The Healing Power of Spices

Healing Yourself Naturally with Spices

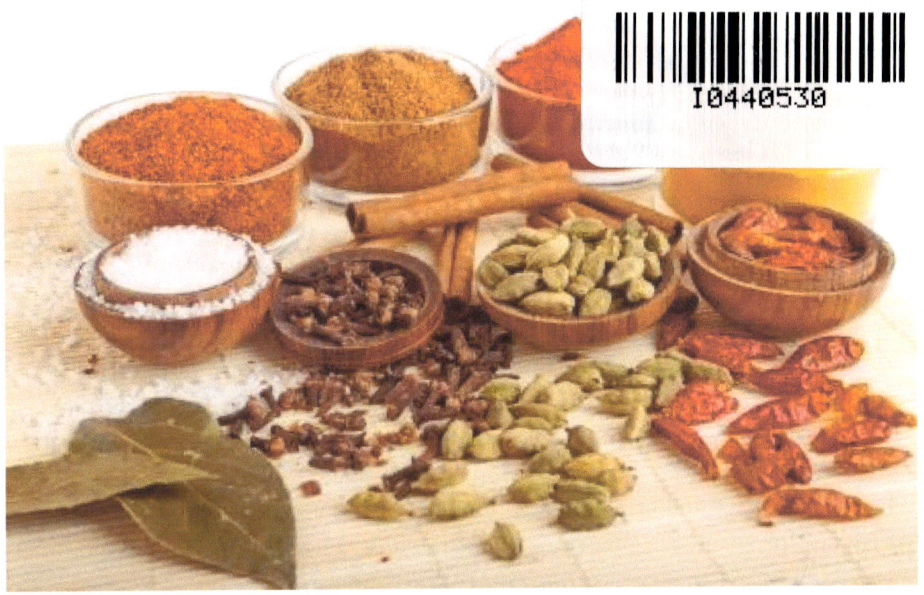

Dueep Jyot Singh

Healthy Living Series

Mendon Cottage Books

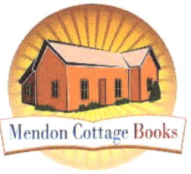

JD-Biz Publishing

Disclaimer

The information is this book is provided for informational purposes only. It is not intended to be used and medical advice or a substitute for proper medical treatment by a qualified health care provider. The information is believed to be accurate as presented based on research by the author.

The contents have not been evaluated by the U.S. Food and Drug Administration or any other Government or Health Organization and the contents in this book are not to be used to treat cure or prevent disease.

The author or publisher is not responsible for the use or safety of any diet, procedure or treatment mentioned in this book. The author or publisher is not responsible for errors or omissions that may exist.

Warning

The Book is for informational purposes only and before taking on any diet, treatment or medical procedure, it is recommended to consult with your primary health care provider.

Our books are available at

1. Amazon.com
2. Barnes and Noble
3. Itunes
4. Kobo
5. Smashwords
6. Google Play Books

Download Free Books!

http://MendonCottageBooks.com

Table of Contents

Introduction

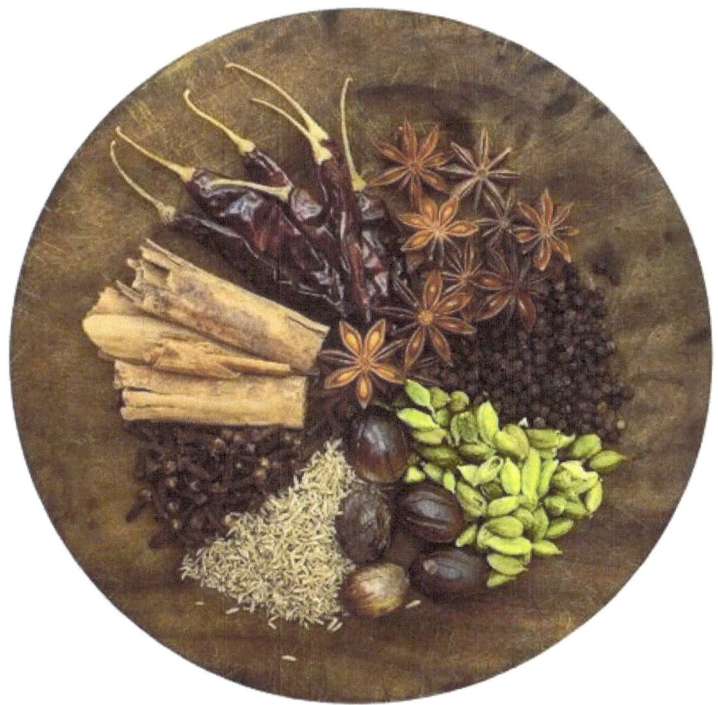

For many decades, I was under the impression that spices were only used as a culinary addition to make a supposedly bland and boring meal delicious. It was only when I began to get interested in naturopathy and natural cures, that I began to see that many of the knowledgeable and experienced naturopaths with whom I came in contact used some spices in some form or the other in order to produce a permanent cure of many ailments.

This book is going to tell you about a large number of spices, and how you can use them effectively to cure yourself in timeworn and time-tested manners.

In ancient times, cooks were highly experienced and knowledgeable healers. They knew all about the effect of spices on the human body as well as how they would affect a particular bio physiological makeup of one particular person. That is why, in Japanese, Korean, and in other countries in South Asia, the cooks were given the duty to heal an ailing person with the food they gave him.

Spices not only add that bit of extra piquancy to our food, but they also provide an equilibrium between the energy given to the body from the normal food intake eaten at every meal and the body's natural bio physiological makeup.

In ancient times, spices were so valuable that any country which produce a large number of spices was considered to be the richest and most desirable of all lands to conquer. The Roman soldiers were given their daily salary in salt – salarus-which they used in making their meal with Garum – anchovy or fish paste , onions and garlic.

I remember an adventure story, where a group of adventurers went out to seek the buried treasure of an Elizabethan sea dog, found the treasure chests after a large number of trials and tribulations and the villains snapping at their heels, and open them up eagerly. Only to find no jewels or pieces of eight, but a large number of spices.

Those spices would have made them multimillionaires in Elizabethan England, but in today's world, they are available on each and every departmental store shelf and in great abundance.

We are fortunate in that way that we do not have to dole out tiny little portions of spices in order to add zest and spice to our food, while waiting for a ship load to come in with their exotic and expensive cargo.

These spices came from the island of Zanzibar and other countries of Africa, India and other tropical countries, where they grew in abundance and were shipped globally since ancient times.

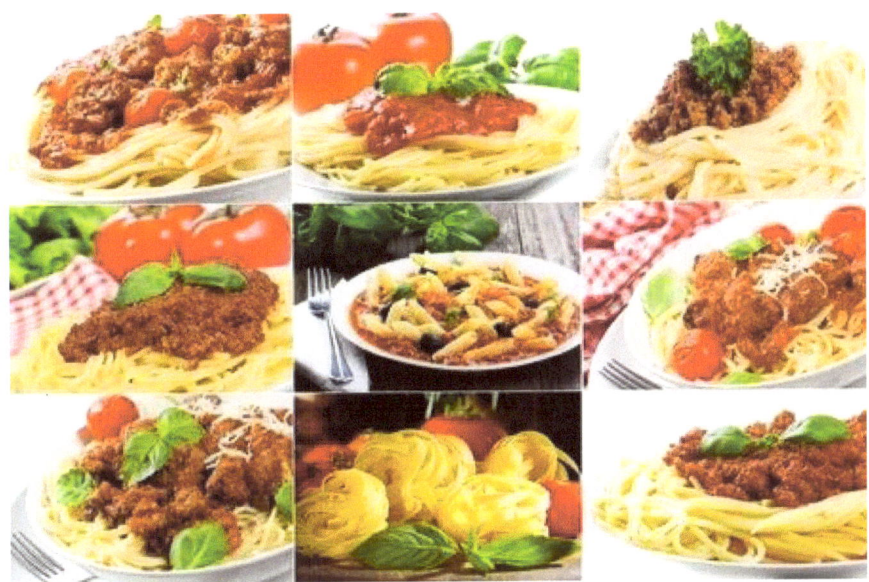

Just imagine these dishes without any spices or salt...

Many of us subconsciously put many of these spices in our foods, not knowing or bothering to understand the reason why they have been added to our diet. These are natural healers and their presence in our food is going to provide us with natural minerals, and other healing elements which are going to keep us healthy, happy and long-lived.

Pepper

It is a historical fact that a Roman Emperor captured aching of one of these islands, and ransomed him by making him kneel on the floor of his court. After that the captured king had to be covered with peppercorns, in order to go free. These are the same peppercorns which we sprinkled with such a liberal hand all over our breakfast, bacon and eggs, soup, or any dish, to which we want to add a little more zest, flavor and piquancy. But then familiarity breeds contempt.

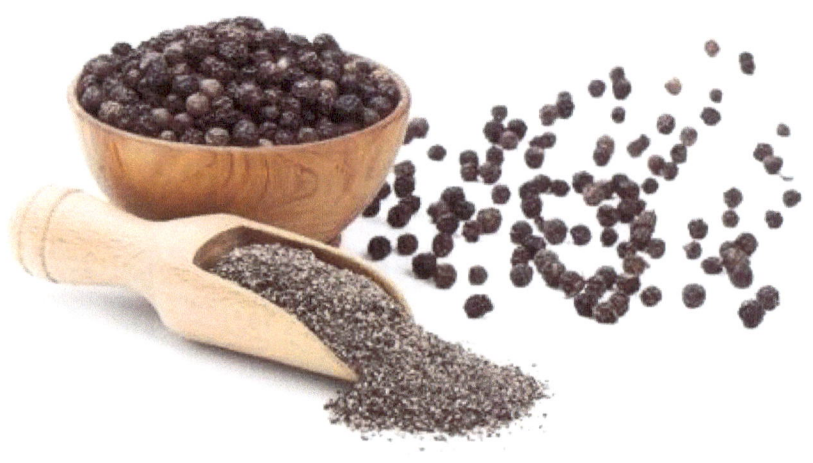

Pepper grows on a climber, which needs the support of a tree in order to grow. The leaves of the pepper vine are spade shaped. The upper portion of the leaf is light green in color while the lower portion is darker green.

There are normally two types of peppercorns found in the world, and the gardeners call them the male vine and the female vine. Both of them have a different appearance from each other. Pollination is normally done through the wind. The peppercorns are around in shape. They are green when they are all, but as they dry up and grow more mature, they turn brown and then black in color. Maturity also brings about more spiciness.

White pepper is just basically black pepper, which has been washed so many times that the peppercorns turn white. These are normally sprinkled on a number of soups and salads, so that the surface of the food is not flecked with tiny black particles and thus spoiling the attractive appearance.

Singapore, and Malaya as well as other South Asian countries is where you can get peppers growing native. It is from here, that they have been spread all over the world by sailors and traders. It is considered to be a stimulant to help heal your heart, kidneys, urinary tract and digestive system, when eaten in small quantities. However, eating peppercorns in large quantities means that you are going to be suffering from stomachache, nausea, and a burning sensation in the urinary passages.

Toothache

People suffering from toothache just need to grind up a few peppercorns, and make the powder into a paste with water. Apply this paste to the affected area and you are going to find your toothache disappearing in a few minutes.

Wounds and Insect Bites

Infections and wounds were treated in olden times by making up a mixture of honey, vinegar and peppercorns, when there was no turmeric around, and applied on the affected area. This would get rid of any sort of infection. It was also supposed to be an effective antidote for insect bites like bee stings, wasps' stings, etc.

In fact, I found this very effective a couple of days ago when I found myself bit by a spider. Normally, when you are bit by a spider, that blistered area turns black, and begins to look like a mole. I applied a mixture of vinegar and powdered peppercorns to counteract the venom of the spider and that blister has nearly disappeared today.

Headaches

This is one remedy, I learned quite recently and I am passing it on to you, so that you never ever suffer from any headaches ever again. Wish I had known it earlier, because then I would not have been suffering from any sort of tension headaches, stress headaches, migraine, or even fatigue headaches, all this while.

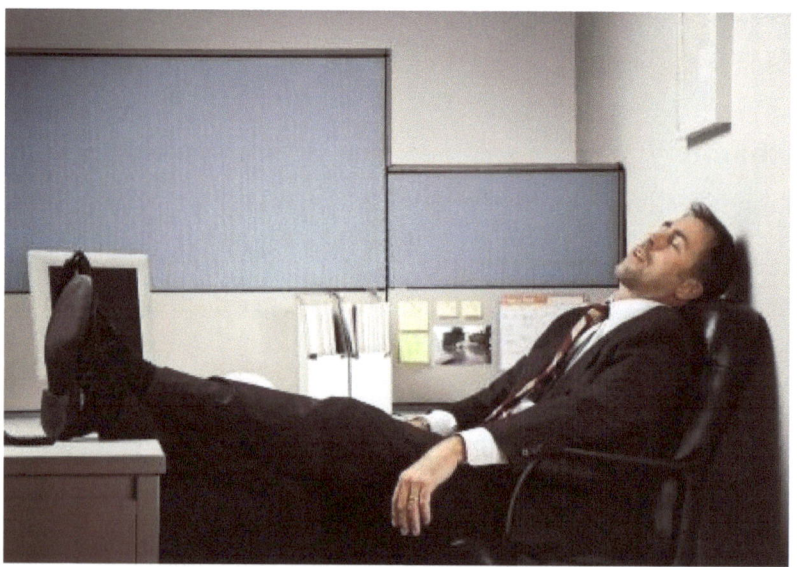

If only I could sleep off this tension headache and relax a bit...

Just take some onion juice and mix it with a little bit of salt. After that, and a little bit of ground peppercorns and mix it to this mixture. Apply it all over the affected area from temple to forehead. This is going to get rid of your headache within half an hour.

Pepper oil is normally used as a massage oil to get rid of gout. Take very small quantities of this oil, before massaging, because it is a strong massaging oil. It is then going to be warmed and then allowed to cool, before you apply it in more quantities all over the affected area. You may also want to try it to make arthritis affected limbs more flexible.

Bishops Weed

The small pungent seeds of *Trachyspermum ammi* are not only a good culinary addition to a number of Eastern dishes, but their "hot" nature makes them a good digestive as well as a preventative for flatulence.

These plants are normally 4 feet high with small leaves. These leaves resemble those of the soil plant. The flowers are small, white and attractive, and each flower is going to ripen into a bishop weed fruit. The seeds inside the fruit are gathered to obtain the spice and use it for either cooking or for healing. They are so tiny, that one cluster of flowers can produce millions of seeds.

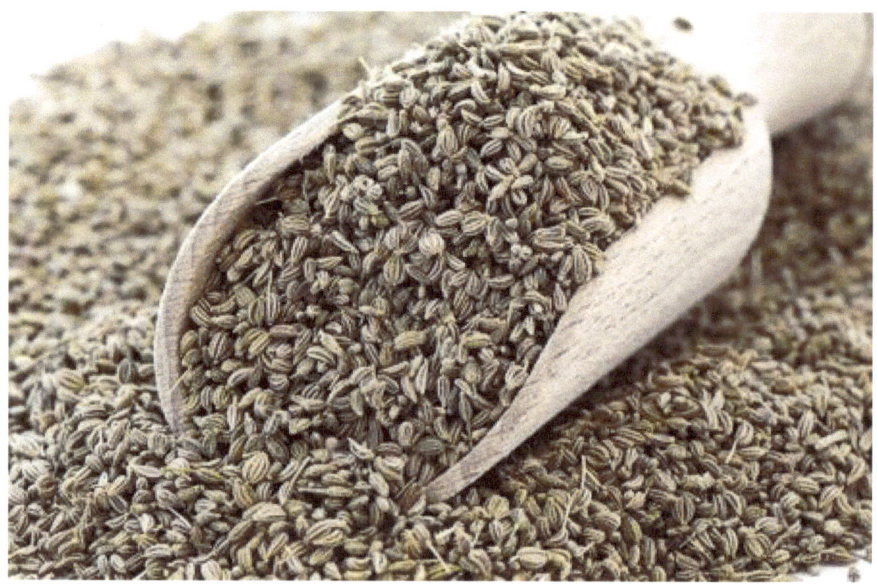

Bishops weed is not very common in the West as a culinary spice, because it is sharp and pungent to the taste. In fact, in ancient medical treatises, bishops weed was considered to be as hot as pepper, as bitter as quinine and as powerful as asafetida to get rid of any stomach ailments.

Naturally, the taste is not bitter, as you would expect from quinine, but the moment you put a little bit in your mouth, it is immediately going to pucker, the moment it feels the sting. The sting is going to go away in a few seconds, but it is very powerful when it is showing its affect.

In the Indian subcontinent, especially when cholera epidemics were universal, and were expected every year, with the coming of the rains the old women of the house managed to protect the youngsters by feeding them lots of bishops weed. This prevented infections, and also got rid of any possible present infection in the body. Naturally, cholera has nearly disappeared from many parts of the earth, today, but any sort of epidemic if occurring can be prevented and cured with these seeds.

Coughs and Colds

My grandmother swore by it, especially in the winters when we used to regularly come down with nasty cough and colds, living in a cold mountainous area.

We were immediately given a handful of bishops weed seeds with a bit of solid peppercorns, and we were told to chew it slowly, without swallowing them. Five minutes of masticating the mixture like a contented bovine, and we would immediately begin to find relief in our coughs. To get rid of the cold, she used to add this mixture to hot milk, and make us drink it down.

And that is how we got rid of any potential chest infections, especially in the winter when our immunity system was not going very strong.

Also, these seeds are an extremely good detoxifying medium. The more you eat them, the more you are going to find your system clearing, especially if you suffer from constipation.

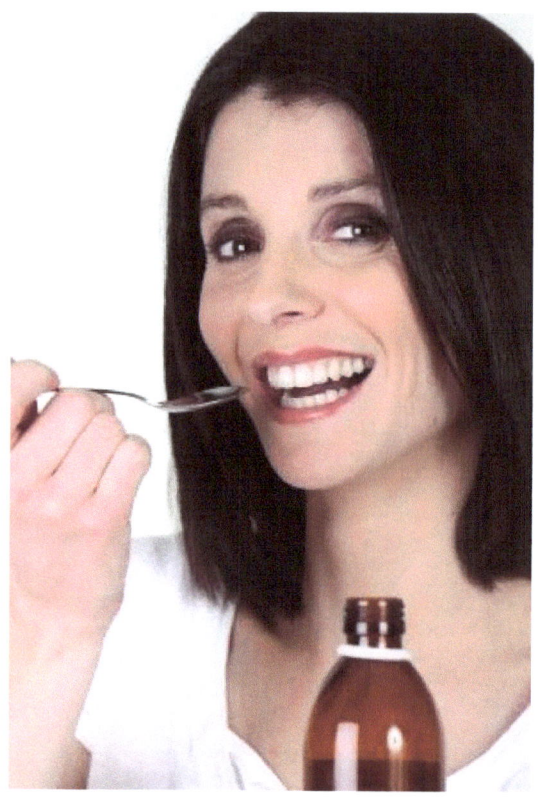

Do not take any cough mixture for cough. Take bishops weed instead and cure yourself naturally.

In fact, in ancient times, half of the stomach problems, urinary infections and chronic cough was cured with the help of a small handful of Bishops weed – about 3 teaspoons –chewed very slowly and then drunk down with warm water.

Bishops Weed Oil

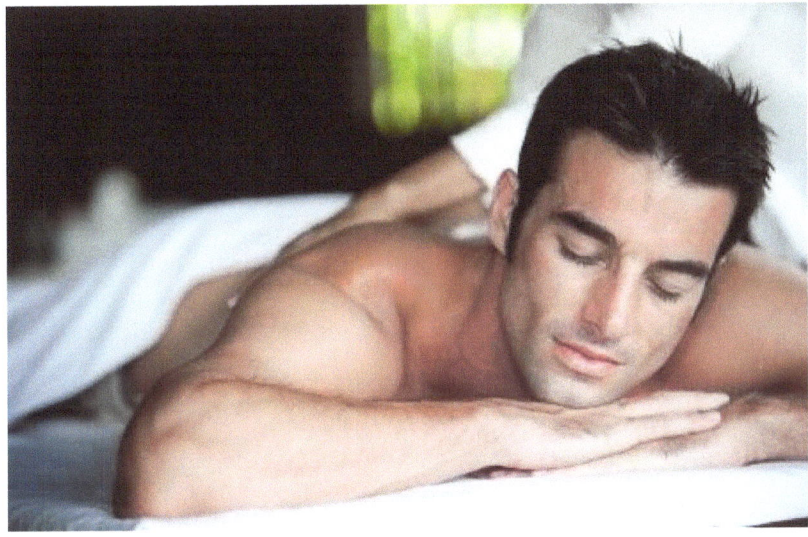

Bishops weed oil is an extremely good massage oil for people suffering from asthma, chest infections, cough, and other chest related problems. Just rub a little bit of bishops weed oil on the chest, for a speedy cure.

In the same manner, it is extremely good for getting rid of any sort of infection in wounds. As in the East, it has been taken for granted that any seed is going to be turned into oil, whenever possible, and that oil used for medicinal purposes, since ancient times, this oil is also taken out, and put in small glass bottles.

The moment you cut yourself, just dab a little bit of this oil on the wound after cleaning it out. I have not used chemical-based antiseptics for the past two decades, like Savlon. If I do not have neem oil and honey to cure my scratches and cuts, I see if I have some bishop weed oil around. It does just fine.

Coriander

Coriander leaves, as well as coriander seeds have long been used as a delicious addition to your food as well as curative natural medicines. Coriander seeds have been since ancient times known to be a diuretic, digestive, preventer of infections and nausea, cough, respiratory problems, and even a cure for lisping and stammering!

Green coriander leaves are fragrant and that is the reason why, a number of the spicy dishes you eat in Eastern cuisine are always sprinkled with onions, pieces of lemon, and chopped green coriander leaves as garnishing.

That is because coriander is excellent to get rid of digestive problems, especially if the dish is very rich and just swimming in hard to digest fat and spices. It also prevents throat infections, and boosts up your digestive system.

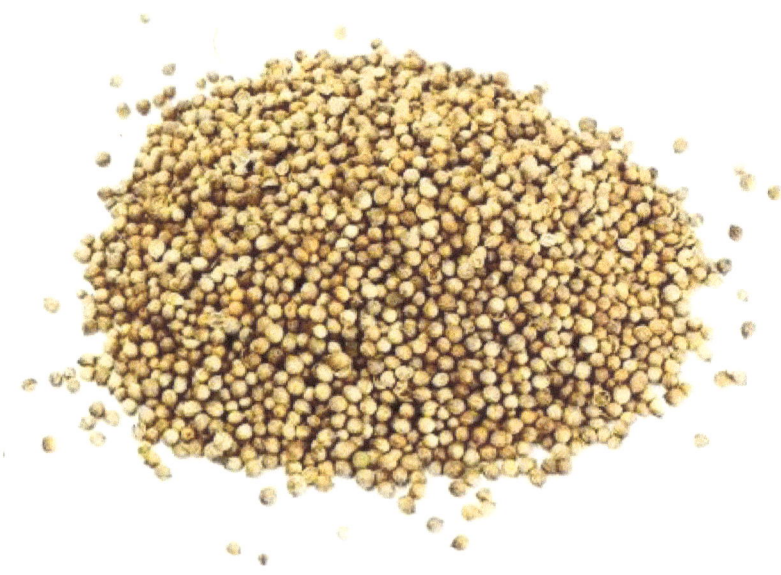

Sprains

I normally apply a mixture of mustard oil, and turmeric with a teaspoonful of honey on any sort of sprains I have, and thus help cure them within the next two days. Along with this, I drink a glassful of hot milk with a teaspoonful of raw turmeric added to it, so that the system can be healed internally. But one fine day I found myself with a painfully sprained ankle and absolutely no milk and turmeric around. You would not have it in a trekking camp.

 But the cook had some coriander leaves, because he could not do without it, and without onions! I just ground them up with a little bit of onion juice and breakfast oatmeal flour and made a paste. Then I applied this bandage to the sprain and by next morning, I was fit to march miles.

When my fellow trekkers asked me where I had learned this trick, I told them that it was just by chance! Actually, I can admit that I was just showing off. I knew that coriander leaves had cooling properties. The onions were antiseptic and both would cool down the inflamed sprained tissue. The flour was just to make a paste of the ground leaves and ground onions and onion juice. But hey, it worked!

Flatulence Cure

Coriander oil, just like mint oil is excellent to get rid of flatulence. Just add two drops of the soil to a glassful of milk before you go to sleep. Your system is going to be cleared by the time you wake and you are not going to suffer from any sort of flatulence brought about by eating indigestible foods.

If you are suffering from stomach ache, you can massage the affected area with a little bit of warm coriander oil. It is also good as a gout massage.

Cumin Seeds

Cumin seeds and cumin oil.

I just cannot do without cumin. In fact, every time I go into a restaurant, I see the amount of cumin seeds, they have added to the dish, and if they have done so with a liberal hand, I know that the cook appreciates the quality of the food which he is making for his clients. Cumin is an essential ingredient, put in rice in many parts of the world, even today.

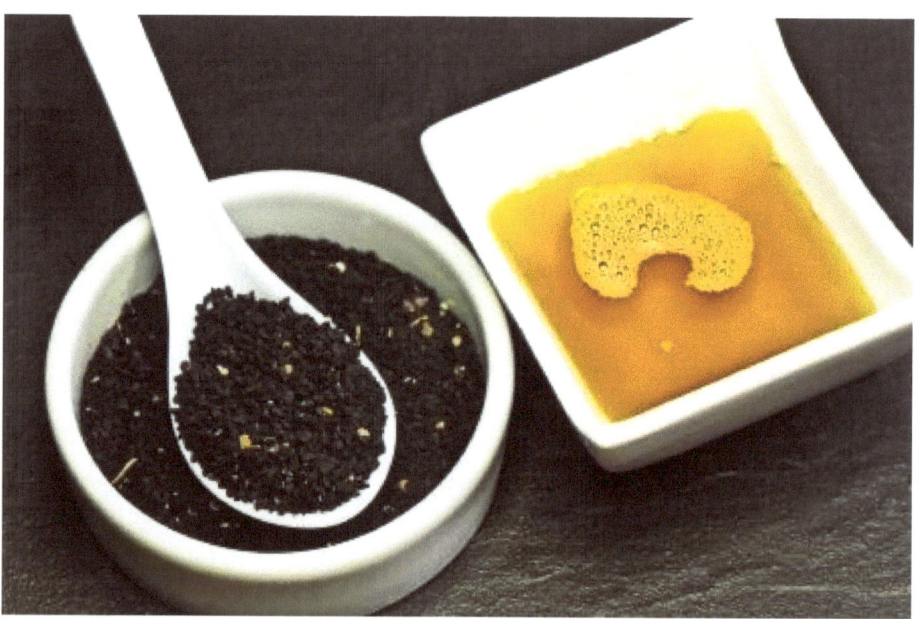

Digestive Water

When I was young, and living in South India, I loved drinking the water from our neighbor's copper water utensil. It had a really nice and delicious taste, which somehow was not found in the drinking water present in our house. It was only later that I found that that lady used to boil up two tablespoonful of cumin seeds, with that day's quota of drinking water for the family every morning, and put them in copper drinking utensils.

The children were not allowed to drink from the fridge or directly from the tap. And they were the healthiest children I had ever seen, even though being often in my company, they ate all sort of occasionally unhygienic stuff, of which their parents never knew.

So if you are prone to stomach ailments, try this cumin water cure for a couple of days. You are going to find yourself rid of all sort of stomach afflictions and infections really soon.

There are two types of cumin seeds found in the market today – white cumin and black cumin. Both types are warming in nature, light to digest and spicy. They are excellent for your brain, eyes, concentration, and curatives for fever, cough, flatulence, nausea, and dyspepsia.

Urinary Infections

People suffering from urinary infections should boost up their cumin water consumption for curing the infection from inside and cumin seeds for a natural healing process.

Cumin for Female Health

Let me tell you some information, which was I overheard spoken by an old relative who being old did not bother much about conventions and modesty, when she was talking about natural processes and earthy matters. She was encouraging her daughter to feed her teenage granddaughter plenty of cumin seeds, so that she had a voluptuous bust! This is one secret, which is definitely going to be well appreciated by all those ladies who are trying to get a Dolly Parton sized bust, because it is supposedly so appealing.

Incidentally, that girl soon developed such a huge bust, that everybody at college called her The Jersey Cow. When I told all my friends, that it was because of cumin seeds, the cumin seed intake in that particular year went up by about hundred percent!

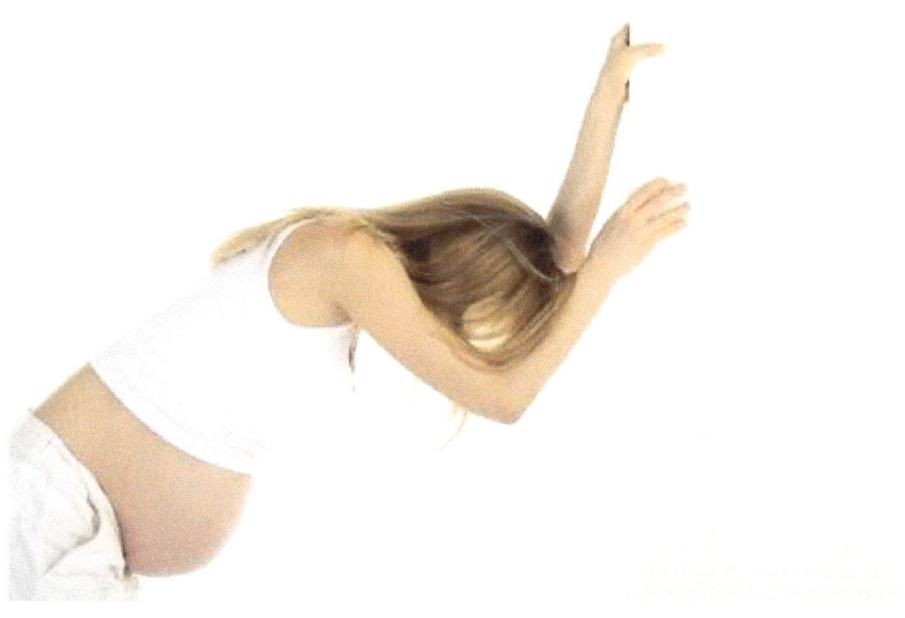

Also, in ancient times, an expectant mother was given a strong decoction of cumin seeds after she had undergone labor. This would clean up the system of any possible infection, increase the quantity of milk in the breasts and also contract the uterus naturally, after the baby was born.

In the same way, women who had problems in their monthly flow were given a decoction of cumin seeds in order to get the system moving naturally again. The seeds keep the female reproductive system healthy and that is why it is considered to be a "Female" herb by ancient herbalists.

Edema

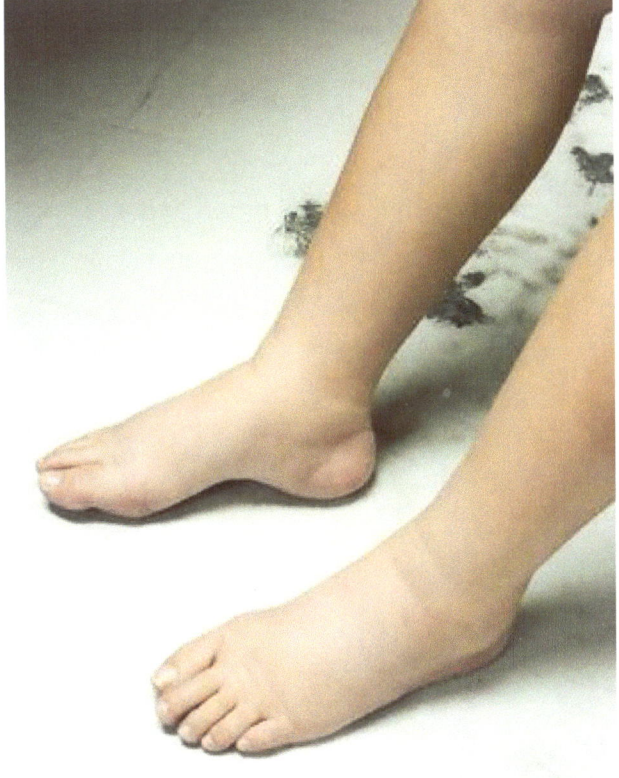

This is rather common at the end of the day...

Edema is normally caused through keeping your feet down on the earth, for a long while, especially if you have been sitting in front of the computer without moving throughout the day.

So the moment you get home, you are going to put your feet in a bucket full of warm water with a little bit of salt and a little bit of mustard oil added to it. This is to get rid of the swelling. After you have soaked your feet for 20 minutes, you are going to put them up at an angle of 90° in the air, to get rid of the swelling and have your ankles coming back to their normal attractive shape.

However, if you do not have mustard oil or salt or hot water, but you do have cumin seeds, just grind them up in a paste and apply them all over the swollen area. This is going to get rid of the swelling. You may try this out in sprains too.

Fenugreek

Fenugreek leaves and fenugreek seeds – both of them are excellent to keep you healthy. These plants are grown globally, and you can find acres of them with one feet high plants with round and sharp smelling leaves. Fenugreek seeds grow in a pod which is about 3 – 4 inches long. The seeds are mustard in color square in shape and 8 to 10 to a pod.

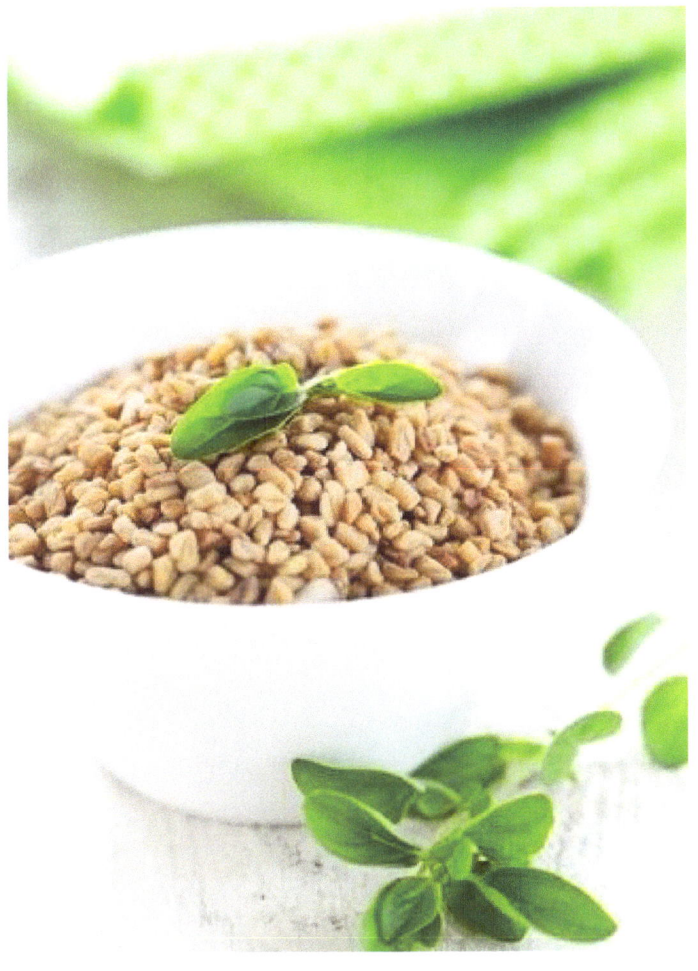

Fenugreek cooked as a vegetable is acclaimed universally and it has been a major part of mankind's diet since ancient times. It is easily digested and cures plenty of stomach problems including dyspepsia and flatulence as well as constipation.

Along with cumin seeds, fenugreek seeds were also given to a mother after labor in a strong decoction to help her heal faster. This helped in the contraction of the womb, after eliminating all the afterbirth tissue and clearing out potentially infective material from the area. In fact, even today, any sort of infection in this particular area is cured by soaking a piece of clean cloth in fenugreek powder solution and inserted in the affected area.

In Taylor Caldwell's Dear and Glorious Physician, the story of Lucanus – the Apostle Luke – she talks about him curing a slave who did not want her child being born a slave and had tried to get rid of it. And this botched up procedure caused her to get infected. She was brought to him, and he cleaned up the affected area with a strong fenugreek seed solution in boiled water. This cured her. So if he knew about this way to cure an infected patient more than 2000 years ago, is it a wonder that even today, fenugreek is being used extensively as an antiseptic and natural cure for female ailments. In many parts of the world, where naturopathy rules supreme , fenugreek seeds and fenugreek leaves are used to keep young mothers healthy.

Fenugreek Seed Balls

Here is a traditional winter ancient recipe, which is normally eaten to get rid of winter aches and pains. It also cures chest infections, cough, cold and flatulence problems.

This is also given to expectant mothers, so that they can give birth to healthy children. This is made up of clarified butter, and that is the reason why it is eaten by old people only in winter because of its warming properties.

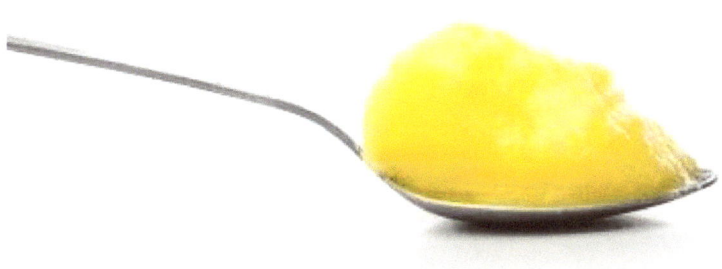

One teaspoonful of clarified butter has enough of concentrated power equal to 4 teaspoons full of ordinary butter and 5 teaspoons full of full cream.

To make up these fenugreek seed balls, you will need hundred grams of fenugreek seeds, half a liter of milk, 250 g of clarified butter, 300 g of flour, hundred grams of Tragacanth gum [more about this particular item later], 2 teaspoons full of dried ginger powder and cumin powder. 30 almonds, 8 to 10 peppercorns, 10 pieces of cardamom, of which the seeds have been crushed lightly and four pieces of cinnamon ground. 300 g of molasses to make up the mixture.

So now, you said that you can get many of these items on your supermarket shelves, but what on earth is Tragacanth gum? Astragalus Gumnifer is an edible gum which has been used since ancient times to provide warmth to an ailing body. It cools you down in the summer, and heats you in the winter![1] but I normally buy it in the winter in order to make these fenugreek balls for the elders of the family.

If you are using sugar, instead of molasses powder it first and then mix it with the rest of the ingredients.

Clean the fenugreek seeds by washing them and leaving them under the shade to dry. Grind them in the grinder to a flour like consistency.

Boil the milk, add this powder to the milk, and let stay overnight the next 8 to 10 hours.

Crush the black pepper, cardamoms, cinnamon and nutmeg into powder. Crush the almonds in little pieces.

Pour the clarified butter in a Wok and fry the fenugreek mixture on low heat until it turns a golden brown in color. You are now going to smell the fragrance of fried fenugreek seeds. Remove and allow to cool.

Take one teaspoonful of clarified butter, and put the small pieces of molasses in the butter. Allow the molasses to melt into a syrup. Now add cumin and ginger powder, black pepper, the almonds, the nutmeg, the cardamom and the cinnamon to the syrup and mix them all together well. Mix the mixture in the molasses syrup.

---

[1] http://www.foodclinic.in/blog/health-benefits-of-tragacanth-gum-gond-katira/

15 g of edible gum Tragacanth is available on eBay USA for USD2.67. You may want to look at more economical sites for the hundred grams needed. Do not use the chemical mixed tragacanth, which is used in the leather industry.

Now you are going to take a fistful of this syrup/fenugreek mixture and shape it into a small lemon sized ball. Make balls until the mixture is finished and place them in the open air for five hours. Your fenugreek seed balls are ready to eat. Reserve them in airtight containers. You are going to eat one in the morning or in the evening with hot milk.

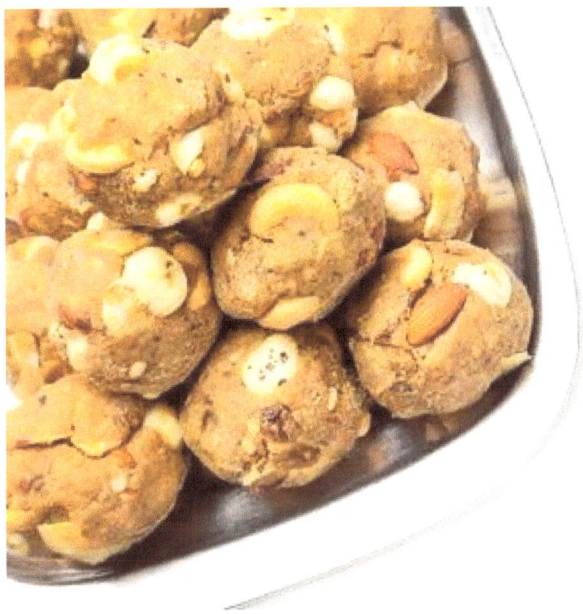

This prevents you from suffering joint pains, aches, arthritis pains and back pains, especially during the winter. You can also add your favorite dry fruits, including walnuts, cashew nuts, pistachio or any other favorite fruits available, to make these balls more edible and tasty.

Cardamoms

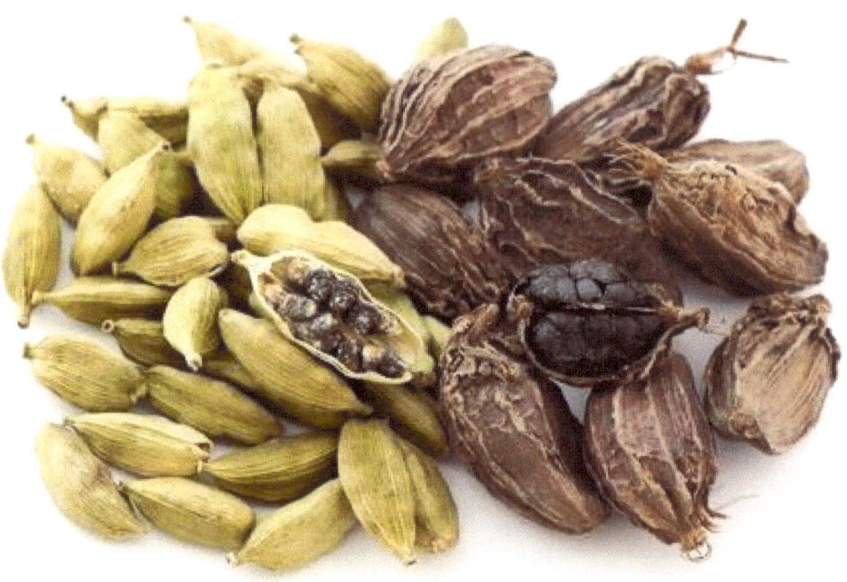

According to ancient medical sciences, cardamoms are light, warm, digestive, and curative for cough, blood problems, asthma, itching, excessive thirst, palpitations of the heart, urinary infections, nausea, and colds.

Excessive Thirst

Now let me tell you how cardamoms cured me of excessive thirst. I am not in the habit of drinking lots of water, unless absolutely necessary. That is the reason why sometimes I go without three – five hours without drinking any water.

This continuous dehydration over a long period of time went up to such a state, that I used to wake up at nights, thirsty as heck, finishing up bottles of cold water in the large thermos flask at my bed side and still feeling thirsty. This happened at least three times a night, which was not healthy for me, interrupting my eight hours necessary sleep.

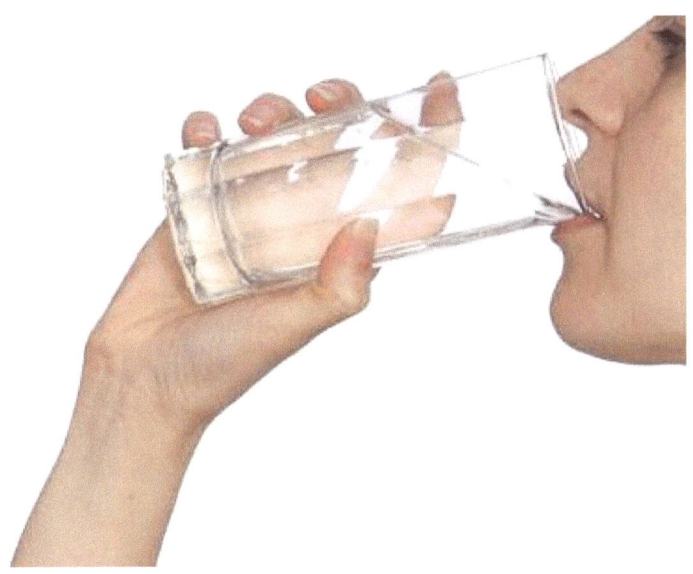

A couple of days ago, I decided to see natural remedies, which would cure me of this excessive raging thirst, apart from drinking lots of water every half an hour. I put two small cardamom pods in my mouth and left them there. I did not bite them for the first 20 minutes, but allowed the saliva to flow naturally into my system. After that I chewed the seeds and the pods for about 20 minutes and then swallowed them. And for the last three days, I have had 10 ours of uninterrupted sleep, without feeling thirsty/dehydrated and wanting lots of cold water in the middle of the night.

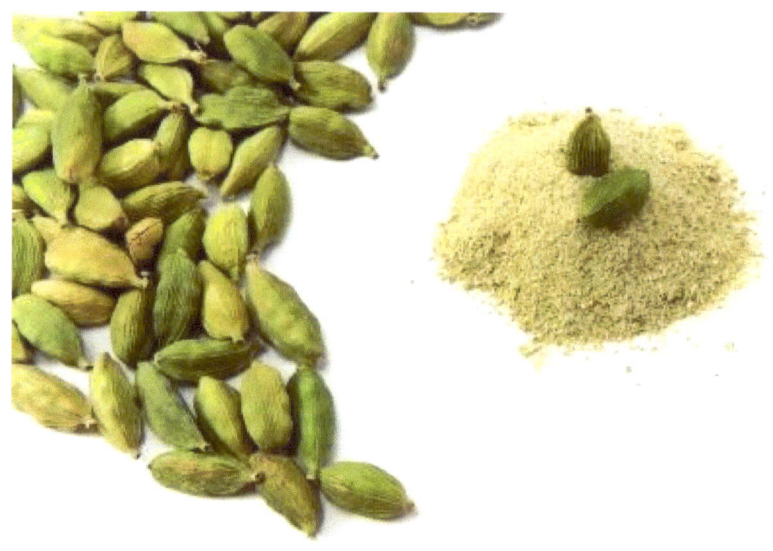

Cardamoms have long been used to sweeten your breath, when you did not have mint around. Pop a few cardamom seeds into your mouth after you have had a meal full of onions and garlic and spices. It is going to freshen your breath. It is also useful to keep your teeth healthy without cavities. Apply some cardamom oil on an aching tooth, if you do not have clove oil available.

If you are suffering from dyspepsia, flatulence, or urinary problems, especially caused by a urinary infection, eat at least two large sized black cardamoms with your meals. Crush the shell lightly so that you can see the seeds. Chew the seeds first. Then chew the shell. This is going to get rid of your stomach problems.

Cinnamon

Cinnamon plants are found commonly in Malabar, Cochin, China, Sri Lanka, Sumatra and Java. Cinnamon leaves are also dried up and used in native medicine, even though we know more about the cinnamon bark. The flowers are red and white in color. They have a sweet fragrance. Cinnamon flowers give a fragrant cinnamon essence, cinnamon water and cinnamon oil.

Cinnamon is normally used for getting rid of swellings since ancient times. In fact, I saw a swelling in the foot being massaged with a mixture of cinnamon powder mixed with clay and made into a paste with water. Apart from this clay mixture, removing all the dirt and grime from the upper surface of the massaged foot, the swelling also went down.

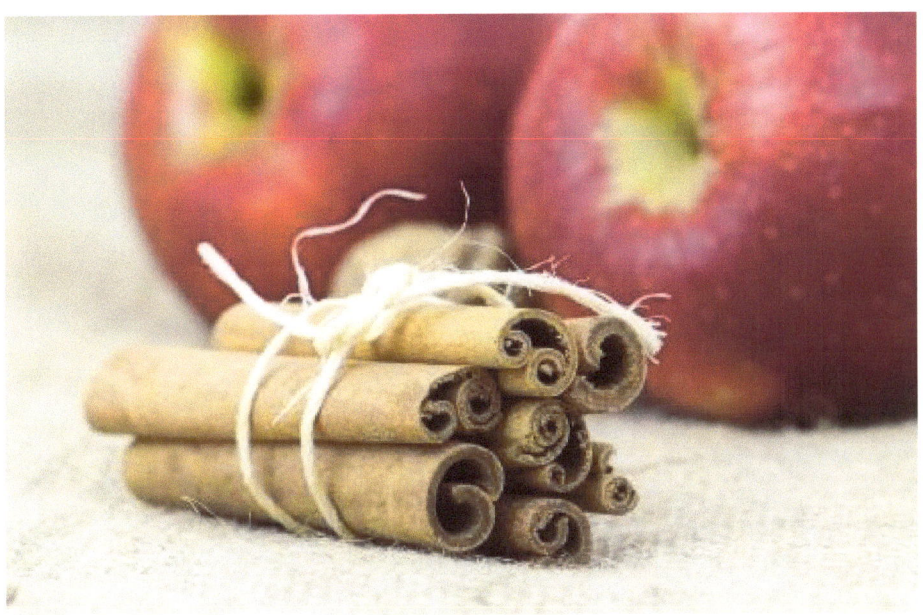

Cinnamon has long been known as an antibiotic. Since ancient times, it has been eaten to get rid of infections in the stomach. In fact, injections of cinnamon extract have been given by naturopaths in order to cure ailments brought about by excessive heat in the body. People suffering from TB are also given injections made up of cinnamon extract. This extract is known as Cinnamic acid.

If you are suffering from any sort of swelling in your mouth or even dental problems, all you have to do is apply a little bit of cinnamon oil to the affected area. It works wonders.

Cloves

Zanzibar was known as the island of cloves, in ancient times, and the marinas knew that they were approaching this island, the moment they felt the fragrance from the trees reach their nostrils, borne on sea winds. Even today, people enjoy visiting this island to see this rich green foliaged tree for fuming the air with its fragrance.

Cloves are the dried flower buds, obtained from this tree. The flowers are harvested, when they are red in color, and plucked by the hands to be dried in the sun. They turn into fragrant black cloves in three days.

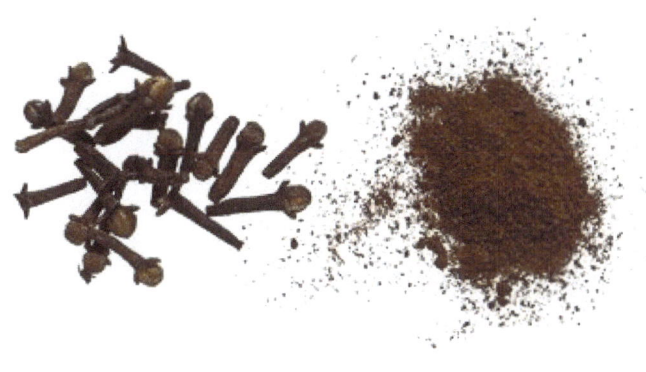

Clove Water

Clove water is made by taking 20 g of fresh cloves – do not powder them – and put them in 4 L of water. Boil on low heat until the quantity is reduced to half. You do not need to filter this. Remove the quantity of the water when needed and as you need it. If you find any cloves coming out with the water, put them back into the airtight glass container.

Clove water is good for rinsing out your mouth, after your meals. You are not going to suffer from any toothache when cloves are around. You can also prevent any cuts from getting infected by just rubbing a couple of pieces of cloves into a paste with water and applying it on the wounded area. This is an excellent antiseptic and healer.

Cloves have been long used since ancient times to get rid of blood infections, cough, asthma and TB. They are also capable of getting rid of dyspepsia, especially when you ate them ground up in your meal.

Cloves for Aches

Everybody knows that clove oil is excellent for getting rid of that persistent nagging tooth ache, which is going to start bothering you late at night when there are no dentists around. If you do not have clove oil, ready at hand, just crush a couple of cloves and mix them with water. Then apply this mixture all over the affected area. This is going to get rid of your toothache.

Also gargle with salt water to get rid of any sort of infection in the gums caused by the toothache.

Clove oil is not only good for toothache, but I have found that it is excellent for headaches, and backache. After all, if it is going to numb the area around your tooth, and get rid of all the pain, why should not it do the same for the aching head or the back? Just warm a little bit of clove oil, and rub that affected area for a couple of minutes. You are soon going to find the ache going away.

My Pain Relieving Mixture

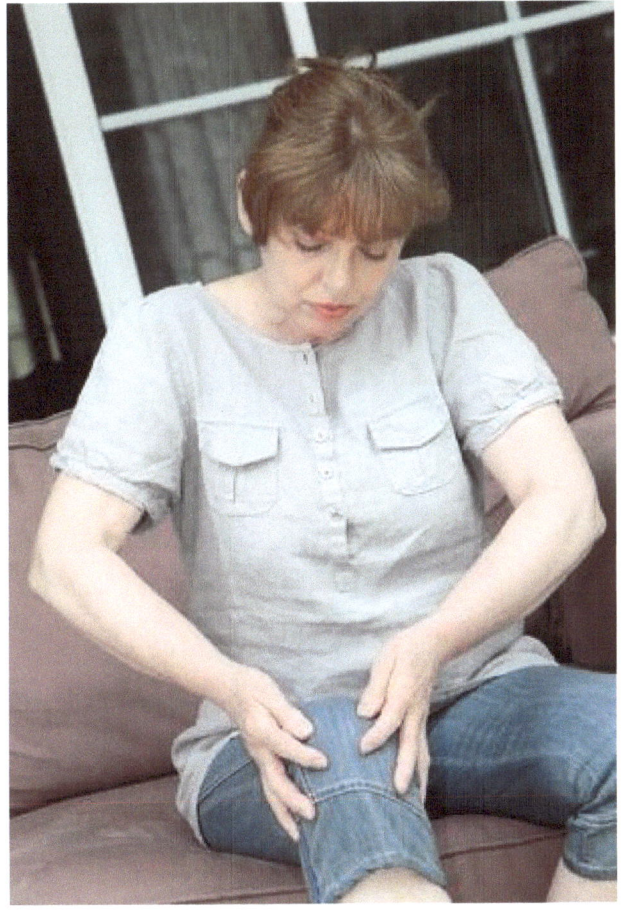

I have made up a mixture of 2 tablespoons each of clove oil, powdered ginger, camphor and eucalyptus oil, one teaspoonful of cinnamon powder and half a teaspoonful of red chili powder. Put them in a bottle after mixing them thoroughly. The moment you suffer from any sort of ache anywhere, especially muscle aches, this does wonders as a massage oil. Do not drink it!

Add the red chili powder if you are using this in winter. If you are using this the rest of the year, do not add the chili powder.

If you want it in an ointment form, use either 10 g of cocoa butter or 10 g of beeswax. Melt it in a container full of water, and then add the ingredients slowly, mixing on a slow fire. When all the ingredients are mixed thoroughly, place to cool, and then shift into your favorite glass jar.

If I want, I can patent this natural medicine as DJ's Panther Balm. It bites like a Panther but takes the pain away!

I use this every evening, when I get up all stiff and sore from sitting on my computer without moving a muscle. And within 15 seconds, I am limber again, not exactly ready to go dancing but able to move without making ooh, aaah and ouch noises. A couple of days ago, I woke up with muscular stiffness, brought about by sleeping in one position, throughout the night, and I just put 2 tsps full of this mixture in about 10 tablespoons full of warm coconut oil. After that, I massaged that area, and allowed the goodness of these spices to seep in for 20 minutes before I went in for my shower.

No stiffness, and I could do lots of dancing, if I wished thanks to the muscle loosening massage.

Cloves For Throat Infections

Here is another natural remedy, which was demonstrated before me, to cure a child suffering from a chronic throat infection. My friend the naturopath just lit a lamp with oil and a cotton wick. After that, she placed a clove in the light of the lamp and ordered the child to inhale the clove smoke. It really got rid of the infection. Apart from this, it left the area perfumed as well, as got rid of any vestiges of bad breath!

In fact I have also made my own personal toothpaste mixing up 2 teaspoons full of salt with one teaspoonful of powdered cloves, half a teaspoonful of powdered alum and cinnamon, and some pieces of powdered neem bark. If you do not have neem bark, you can use 1/8 teaspoonful of neem oil. It is going to give the toothpaste a little bit of a bitter taste, but you can be assured that you are never going to suffer from dental problems, gingivitis, halitosis, or any sort of problems in the teeth or in the gums ever.

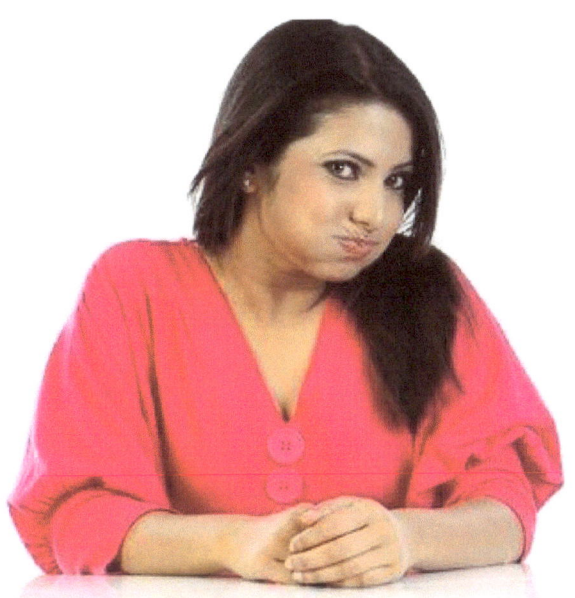

Just swishing clove water around in your mouth can help prevent dental problems and throat infections.

If you do not have cloves at hand, but do have clove oil, use five drops in the mixture. Clove oil is very powerful and too much of clove oil on your gums mean that you are going to be suffering from blisters on the gums instead of a healed dental set.

Cloves are also excellent diuretics and good cures for asthma. So use cloves as painkillers as well as healthy spices in your food.

Ginger

Ginger has long been used since ancient times as a healthy spice as well as a healing agent. Ginger flourishes in areas, where the soil is sandy because it does not enjoy too much of a soggy ground. Soil with plenty of calcium and limestone content is excellent for cultivating ginger. The plant is about 1 ½ feet high. Native Ginger flourishes in mountain areas, also.

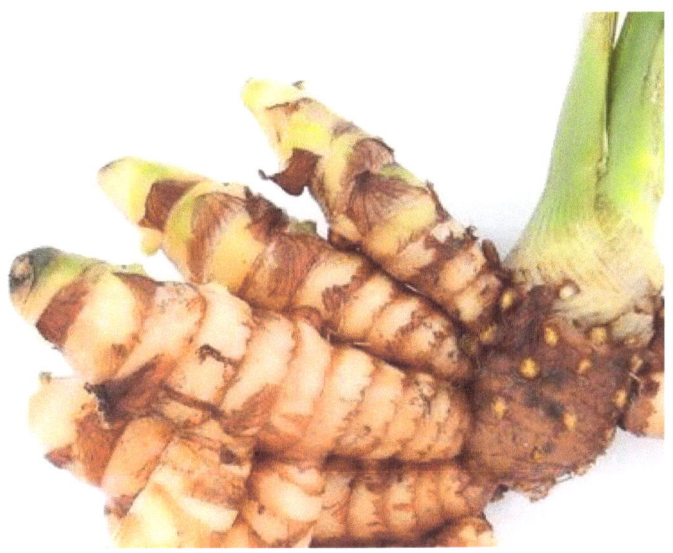

Ginger is warming in nature and constituency that is why it should not be eaten in large quantities in the summer. However, it is the best spice to eat in the winter. It is strong, and heavy to digest, when eaten in large quantities. It is also a good antiseptic.

If you are suffering from acidity problems, you may want to eat a little bit of crushed ginger with salt about 10 minutes before you begin your meal. In many parts of the East, you are going to see a permanent bowl on the table, with a little bit of ginger, vinegar/lemon and green chili peppers placed there to be eaten with each and every meal.

In fact, ginger has been known since ancient times to be an excellent spice to clear up the problems of speech, including lisping and even hoarse voices. The moment you feel your voice getting hoarse, just chew a piece of raw ginger, and allow the juice to soothe your voice.

Incidentally, a couple of days ago I happened to see a video on YouTube, in which a woman was teaching people how to get a hoarse voice. Talk about utter futility. Are there people out there, who considered harsh and hoarse voices to be attractive and sexy? There is one born every moment! Here are people trying to sweeten their voices, and making them more musical an attractive and here are other people teaching people how to make their voice hoarse like as if you are suffering from a cold.

That also reminds me from an utterly useless book. I happened to read a couple of years ago, where the heroine "had a lovely [!] croak like that of a frog "and she kept singing in her hoarse, unmusical voice sounding like the shriek of a cat. And everybody around her thought that polluting of the atmosphere amazingly beautiful. No thanks, I did not. A hoarse voice cannot be lovely. A frog's croak is loud, harsh, unmusical and discordant.

This made me understand that the woman writer who wrote the book had a terribly discordant, ugly, harsh, croaking voice of her own and she was trying to make it appealing to her audience. I shut the book on page 3, when I heard the heroine singing in her quote lovely croak unquote, before she met the tone deaf hero.

So if you do not want to sound like a foghorn suffering from laryngitis, eat lots of ginger.

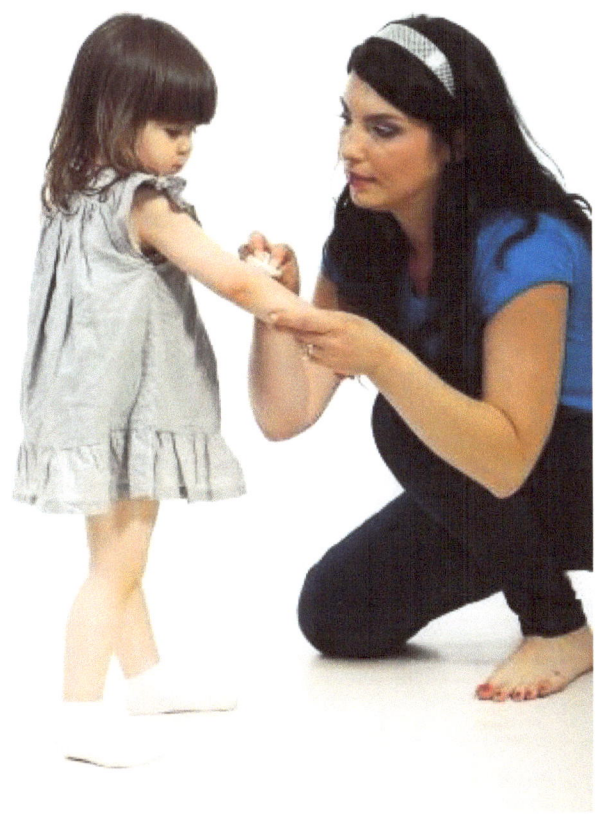

Since ancient times, ginger has been used as an antiseptic to get rid of wounds and infections, especially skin diseases like eczema. If you are suffering from ringworm, just grind some ginger, add some salt and just a little bit of turpentine oil and make a poultice. Apply this mixture, along with the juice to the affected area and bandage it up. The eczema will have vanished within the week.

Ginger Cure for Asthma

There are so many people suffering from asthma and respiratory as well as chest infections all over the world today, and spending millions of dollars on medicines, when they could be cured naturally through ginger.

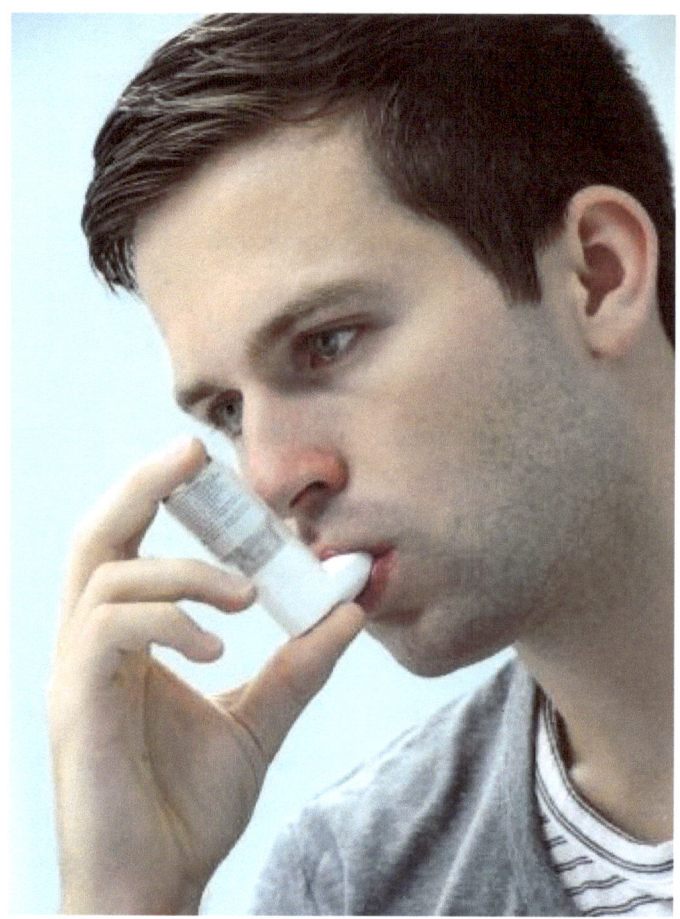

Here is my asthma recipe, which is excellent to get rid of this respiratory ailment permanently. Take 30 g of ginger juice and 30 g of honey. You are going to drink this mixture, three times a day until you are totally cured. If you have a really chronic case of asthma , here is an ancient remedy, which will need a little bit of effort, but it is going to cure your condition completely.

Get some pearl oyster shells and wash them thoroughly. After that, just place them in an earthenware cooking pot over low heat until you get the ashes of these oyster shells. Actually, they are just calcium, but we need the ashes. You are now going to grind the ashes, and do a little bit of filtering, so that there is no solid residue present. Now, you are going to take out 5 g – 1 teaspoon of this powdered oyster shell mixture, and mix it with fresh ginger juice. Make it into a pea-sized ball. The powder should be enough to make 40 of these oyster shell ginger balls.

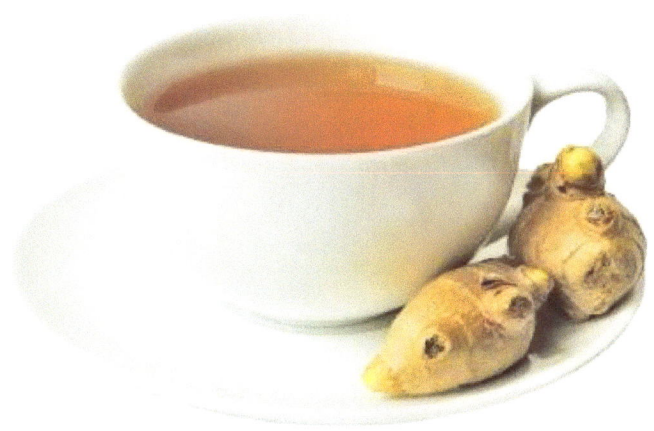

You are now going to eat these, to a day, morning, evening, for 20 days, drunk with ginger tea.

Ginger tea is made easily, by just adding some pieces of ginger to your favorite cup of tea, and allowing to boil for a couple of minutes. You can either throw the ginger pieces away into your compost heap, when you are filtering the tea, or you can chew the pieces of ginger. So you are going to get two doses of ginger tea and ginger pellets every day morning and evening.

20 days – asthma gone completely, even very serious chronic cases. Try it out right now.

Some little pieces of ginger and hey presto, you have ginger tea.

Ginger for Dyspepsia

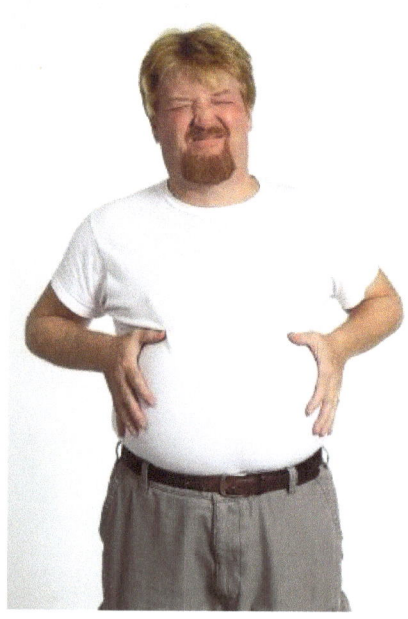

Ginger is excellent for people suffering from stomach ailments, especially dyspepsia. I have also seen that it is useful for those suffering from acidity.

Just add the juice of one lemon into half a cup of ginger juice with a little bit of salt to taste. Sip it slowly, to allow the ginger to work its magic.

If you are suffering from constipation, sip ginger juice and lemon with a little bit of powdered rock salt added, before and after your meal. A couple of days, and no constipation. It will have been cured permanently.

Diarrhea Cure

Even though we as children had a really strong digestive system allowing us to eat all sorts of things without possible side effects, sometimes we fell prey to diarrhea and dysentery because of bad water. That was when we were given a cupful of hot water in which my grandmother had crushed a number of pieces of ginger. We had to sit quietly until the ginger juice had become an infusion in the hot water, and it was ready to drink. And then we had to sip it really slowly. 2 cups of this every day and this cured the diarrhea within a couple of days.

Dried Ginger

Dried ginger is much more powerful than raw ginger and that is why it is used in ginger tea, only as a last resort. You are going to put 1/8 dried ginger powder, in about 4 cups of water, when you are concocting a powerful healing infusion.

Dried ginger is normally made by rubbing pieces of raw ginger roughly. This gets rid of the upper covering. This ginger is then washed and dried in the shade.

Dried ginger is fragrant, and heat producing. That is why it is drunk mainly in winter, because the moment you drink it, you are going to feel a sort of warmth spreading out from your stomach to the rest of your body

Red Chilies

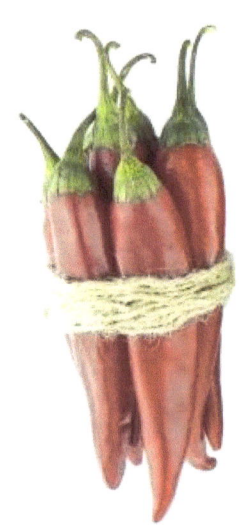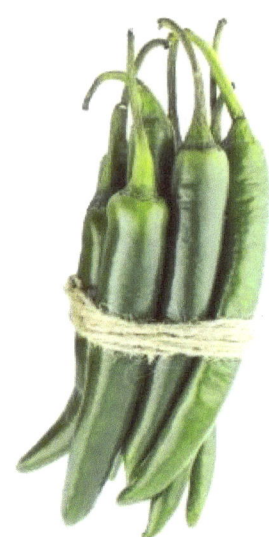

There are a number of chilly varieties available all over the world, from round globular heart varieties, to long elongated miser varieties. A chilies considered to be heating in nature and if you look through ancient medical treatises in the East, you are not going to find any cures in which chilies have been used. That is because this spice came to the East, later in the game, somewhere around the 12th – 13 century, and within eight centuries, it had become an integral part of the social ethos, culture and cuisine.

In fact, when my brother got married, the sisters of the bride, her guests, and her relatives and her friends kept singing about me as *sister-in-law, red chili.* For a moment I was rather pleased because chilies are known to be hot, no pun intended, until I found out that they meant that I was as quarrelsome and as shrewish as a red chili, in keeping up with the stereotyped role of sister-in-law!

Chilies are never applied raw on the skin, when you are using it as a massage. They are also not eaten in large quantities, because they are going to affect your digestive system and stimulate it into possible stomach problems. People suffering from piles are told not to eat chilies, because they cannot afford any sort of problems in the stomach including stomach ulcers.

Chilies for Alcoholism

In many parts of the country, people suffering from alcoholism and opium addiction are given a mixture of orange juice with aniseed mixed, three times a day. Apart from that, they are given a diet, with lots of chilies in it, because it is seen that the chilies counteract the withdrawal symptoms and the craving for opium and alcohol.

 So if you find yourself wanting to reach for that dry martini yet once again, telling yourself that you can take it and leave it, reach for something with lots of chilies in it, instead. You are going to find yourself craving alcohol lesser as time goes by.

Traditional Winter Hot Oil

This Winter oil is normally made traditionally at the onset of winter, so that the members of the family do not suffer from the cold. They are placed in glass bottles and never in plastic and metal bottles. You are going to take just a little bit of this oil and warm it. Remember, because it has a chilli content in it, it is going to be harsh on your skin for the first few instants, and that is why you are never going to use this on the soft and delicate skin of a child.

25 g red chilli powder

Two tablespoonfuls black pepper powder.

1 tablespoon full dried ginger powder

One powdered clove

2 tablespoons mustard powder

1 ¼ cups coconut oil or vegetable oil

This is originally made in mustard oil, but because mustard oil has a very strong aroma, I am substituting coconut oil. Coconut oil is equally powerful and equally aromatic, but somehow it is more popular with people in the West.

You can prepare this oil in two ways. One is in the summer, when you can put all the ingredients in a bottle filled with oil. Place the bottle in the sun and allow to infuse in the summer heat for about two months. Shake this glass bottle regularly.

But if winter is already here, and you were too busy to make this infusion in the summer, do this the other way.

Put the dried ginger, and the chilli in half of the oil in a container with a tight lid. Put this container in a pan with lid. Fill the pan with water up to 2 inches from the top. Allow it to simmer slowly for about two hours. Do not heat the oil directly because it is going to be burnt. That is why it has to be done through boiling in water.

Allow this mixture to cool. Now add the rest of the spices to the oil, and stir vigorously. Add the rest of the oil and return to the boiling water pan. Add more water to make sure that there is no dearth of it. Two more hours of slow boiling is going to give you a red colored very powerful infused oil. I would suggest you filter it, because any sort of sediment at the bottom of the oil is going to spoil it.

Collect those spices. You may use them in cooking or if you want or you may add some more spices to them, and some more oil, and put them outside in the sun for more infused oil by next summer!

You may find some sediment settling down at the bottom of the pan, after about three months. Remove that sediment or watery liquid which may just be parts of herbs which were not filtered, initially, appearing to settle down at the bottom of the bottle. This is going to spoil the oily if it is not removed.

Remember that the cold months of winter does not mean that you need to suffer. Use a little bit of this oil to massage those aching joints and pains.

Chillies Infused Oil

1 1/2 cups of vegetable oil and 250 grams of chili powder gave me 1 1/2 cups of infused oil.

•   Place half of the Chilli powder and all the oil in a container with a tight lid.

•   Put a container in a pan, fill the pan up with water to within 1 inch of the top of the container and simmer this slowly for 2 hours. This water bath makes sure that your precious oil is exposed to prolonged heating without spoiling the oil by burning or boiling. To save time and energy costs, I normally boil 2-3 airtight containers together.

•   After two hours, allow the mixture to cool slightly and then strain it well. Now, we are just halfway through the process and the infusion has changed color. Refill the canister with the remaining powder, cover with the strained oil and return to the water bath. Simmer gently for another two hours. Don't forget to replace the lid! Also make sure to check the water level to make sure that the water has not boiled away completely. Nobody has any use for burnt oil.

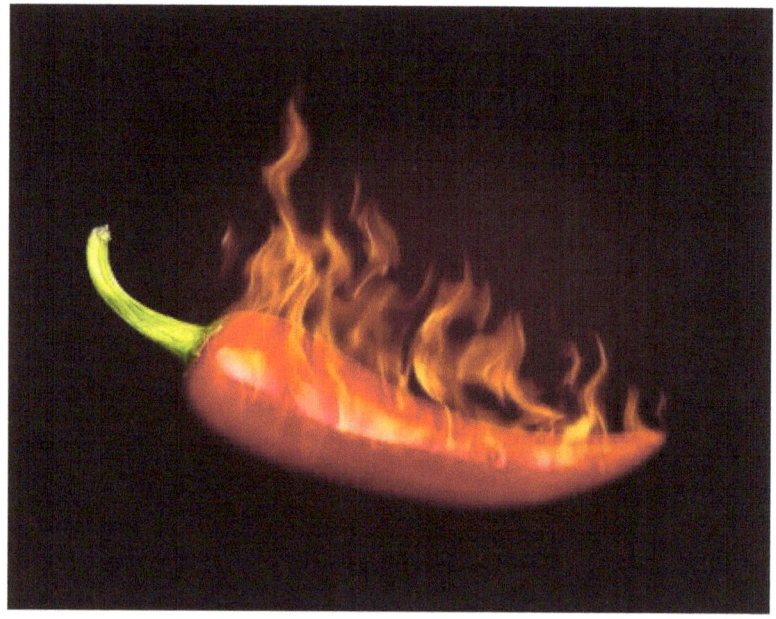

When the oil has cooked enough, pour it through a muslin cloth or very fine strainer. If you are using old powder, there might be some watery liquid at the bottom of the oil. Remember to separate out this liquid and throw it away, because it is quite certain to spoil the oil if it is left unattended.

Once the oil has been strained , gather all the residue in the cloth and wring them out to extract every drop of oil . This oil will keep fresh for a year but it will eventually become rancid. Many cosmetologists thus add some wheat germ oil to delay the spoiling process -- (about 25 g.)

Conclusion

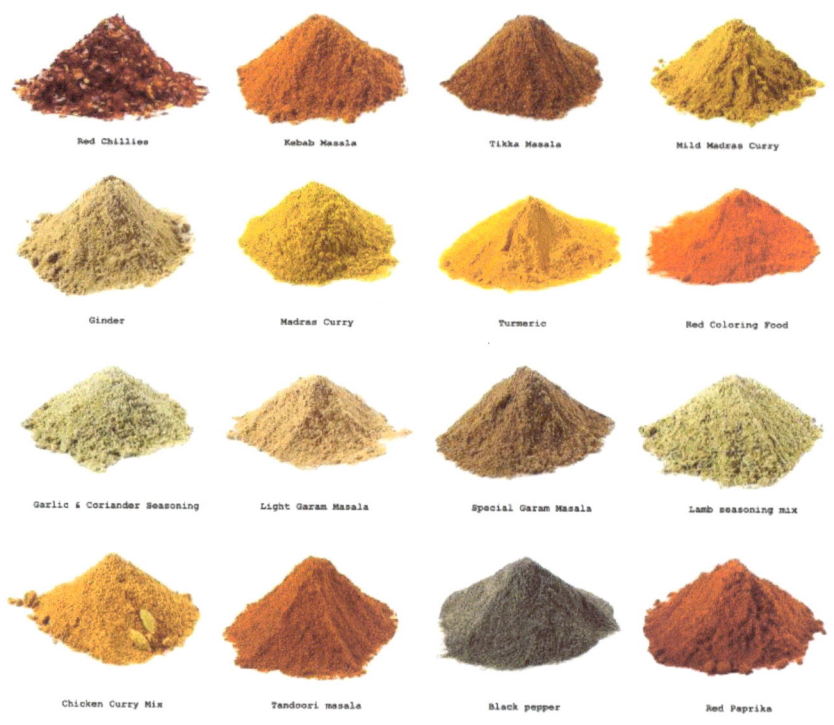

This book has given you lots of information on how spices can keep you healthy. That is why you would like to add the spice content in your food, as well as using them to cure yourself from a number of common natural ailments.

I have not added salt to this book, even though rock salt and sea salt is such a major part of our lives. There are plenty of people in the world, who have decided to eat a salt less diet, thus depriving themselves of necessary and essential sodium. Some of them do not eat it out of sheer stubbornness.

Some may not eat it because of doctors' orders. But even the most stubborn doctor cannot negate the fact that our body needs salt – about 1 ½ teaspoons full each day – in order to keep healthy.

In many parts of the world, salt has iodine added to it, so that people do not suffer from iodine deprivation. Iodine keeps your thyroid working in a proper manner. Iodine deprivation means that you are going to suffer from goiter, hypo and hyperthyroidism.

We as children lived in high mountain and forest areas where we definitely did not get iodine in our food. That is why we grew up with iodine deficiency which means that we have to take tablets every day, providing us with thyroxine. Many of my classmates of that time, also suffer from iodine deficiency, so I can not blame it on genes!

I remember as a child, reading a story about one of these spoilt kings who demanded of his two daughters how much they loved him. The first daughter naturally told him that she loved him more than she loved the sun and the moon and the gods and the king showered her with lands, gifts and other treasures. That daughter naturally turned out to be a greedy mercenary hypocrite at the end of the story. So what is new? The younger daughter, the sweet and lovable one told her father that she loved him as much as she loved salt in her food.

The father was definitely displeased and exiled her. The young princess then managed to go through a large number of adventures, in which she was helped by her friends who she had saved during the adventuring. And then she caught the eye of an Emperor who decided to marry her. So she sent her father and her sister an invitation to the wedding. When her sister came out of her hysterical and jealous fit, she decided to go to her sister's wedding and create some sort of mischief there, for which she was suitably punished at the end of the story being banished by her father and her lands and treasures taken away.

Anyway, here they were, eating delicacies at the wedding feast, but father dear did not seem to be very happy. That was because none of the delicious food had any salt in it.

When the new Empress asked her father why he looked so gloomy and glum, he said that there was something wrong with the food. She said immediately that there was no salt and without any salt, what was the use of eating anything? That is why she had said that she loved him as much as she loved the salt in her food. The father finally woke up and understood the subtle meaning of this statement. And so he showered riches, jewels, and lands over the happy couple who naturally lived happily ever after.

Live Long and Prosper!

Author Bio

Dueep Jyot Singh is a Management and IT Professional who managed to gather Postgraduate qualifications in Management and English and Degrees in Science, French and Education while pursuing different enjoyable career options like being an hospital administrator, IT,SEO and HRD Database Manager/ trainer, movie , radio and TV scriptwriter, theatre artiste and public speaker, lecturer in French, Marketing and Advertising, ex-Editor of Hearts On Fire (now known as Solstice) Books Missouri USA, advice columnist and cartoonist, publisher and Aviation School trainer, ex-moderator on Medico.in, banker, student councilor ,travelogue writer … among other things!

One fine morning, she decided that she had enough of killing herself by Degrees and went back to her first love -- writing. It's more enjoyable! She already has 48 published academic and 14 fiction- in- different- genre books under her belt.

When she is not designing websites or making Graphic design illustrations for clients , she is browsing through old bookshops hunting for treasures, of which she has an enviable collection – including R.L. Stevenson, O.Henry, Dornford Yates, Maurice Walsh, De Maupassant, Victor Hugo, Sapper, C.N. Williamson, "Bartimeus" and the crown of her collection- Dickens "The Old Curiosity Shop," and "Martin Chuzzlewit" and so on… Just call her "Renaissance Woman" - collecting herbal remedies, acting like Universal Helping Hand/Agony Aunt, or escaping to her dear mountains for a bit of exploring, collecting herbs and plants, and trekking.

Check out some of the other JD-Biz Publishing books

Gardening Series on Amazon

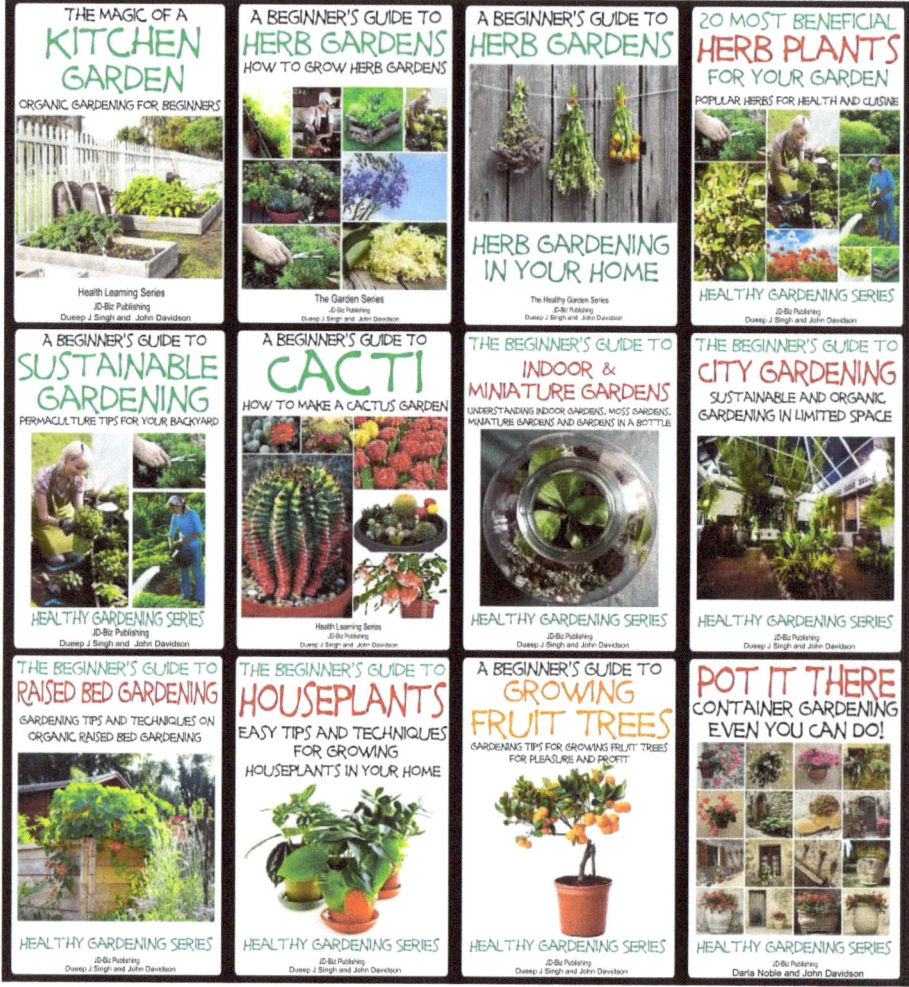

Download Free Books!

http://MendonCottageBooks.com

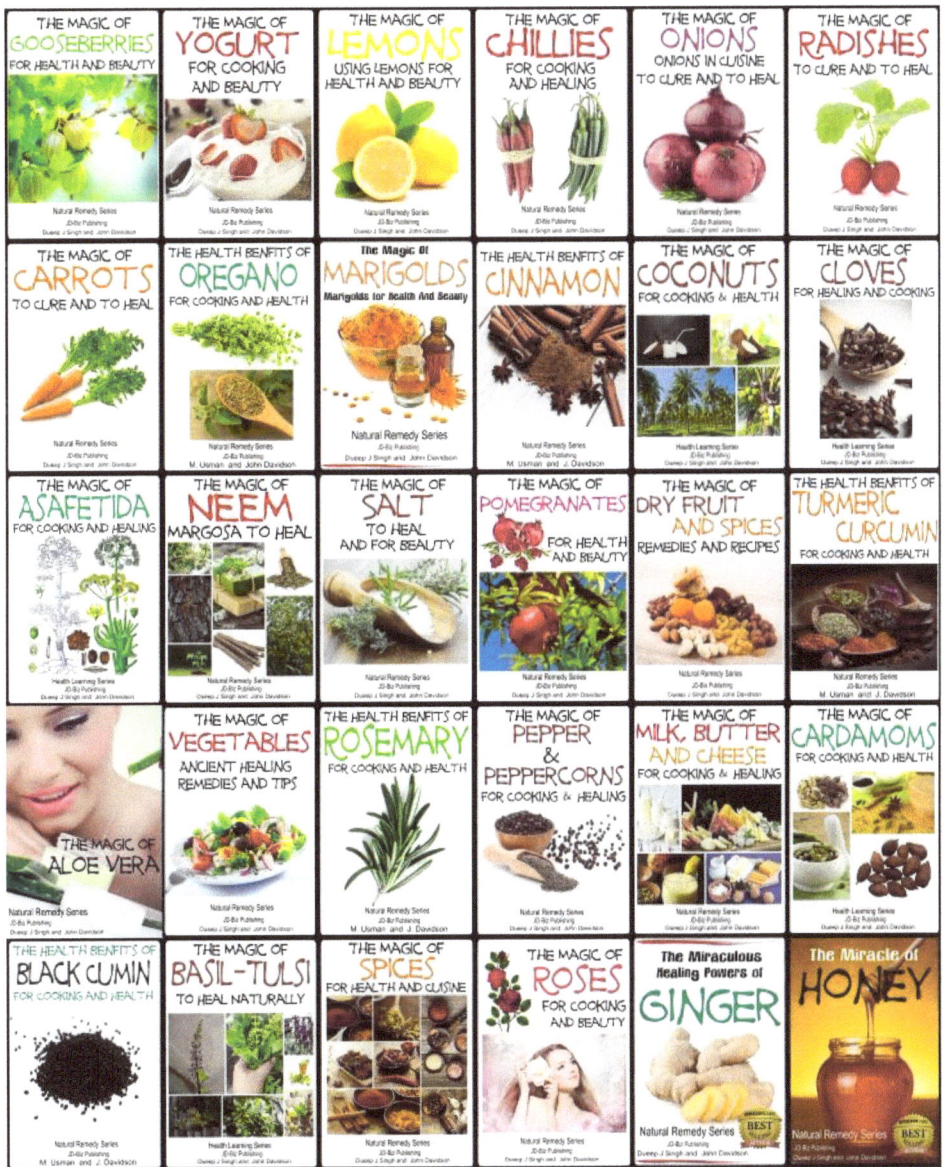

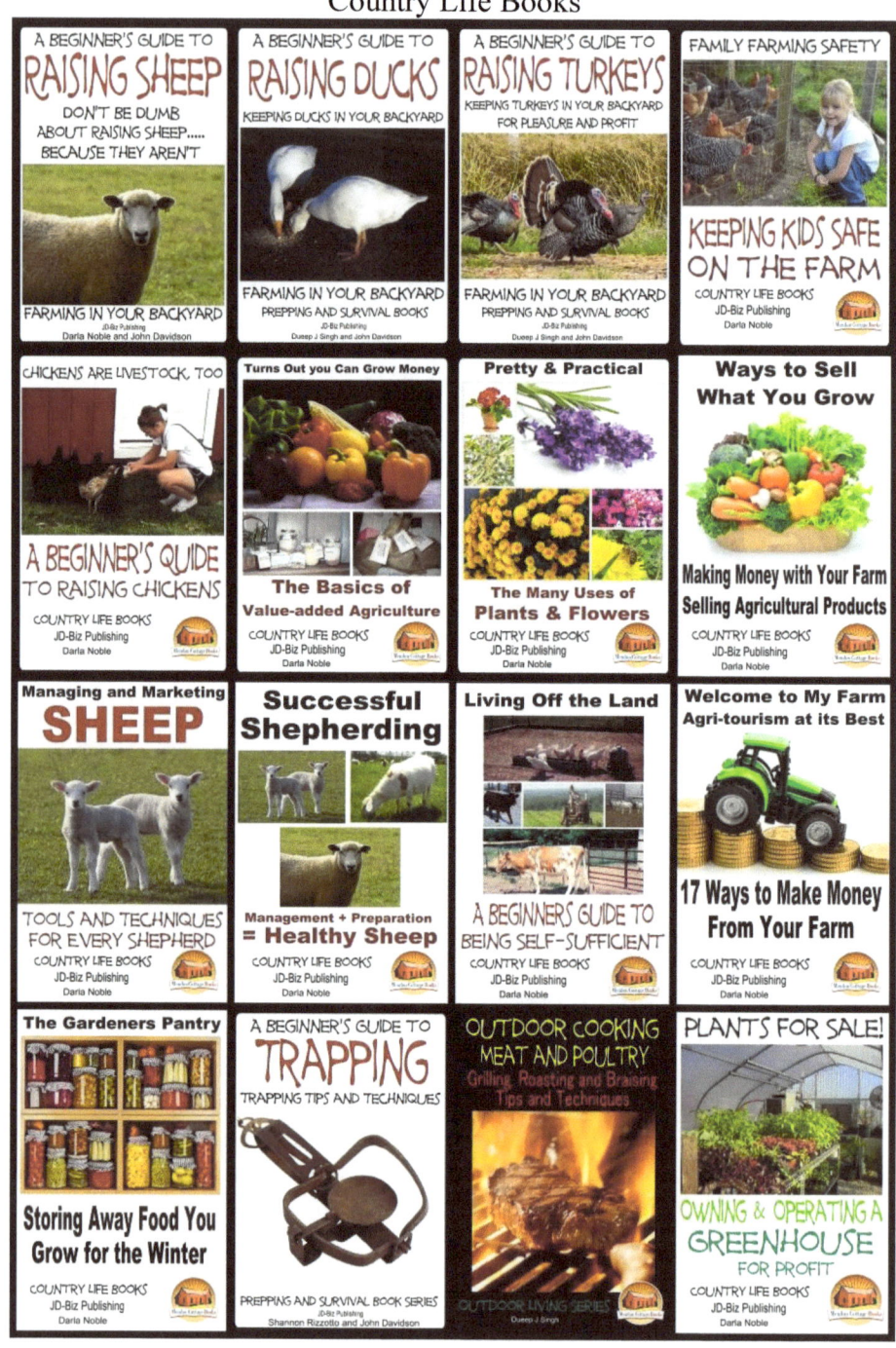

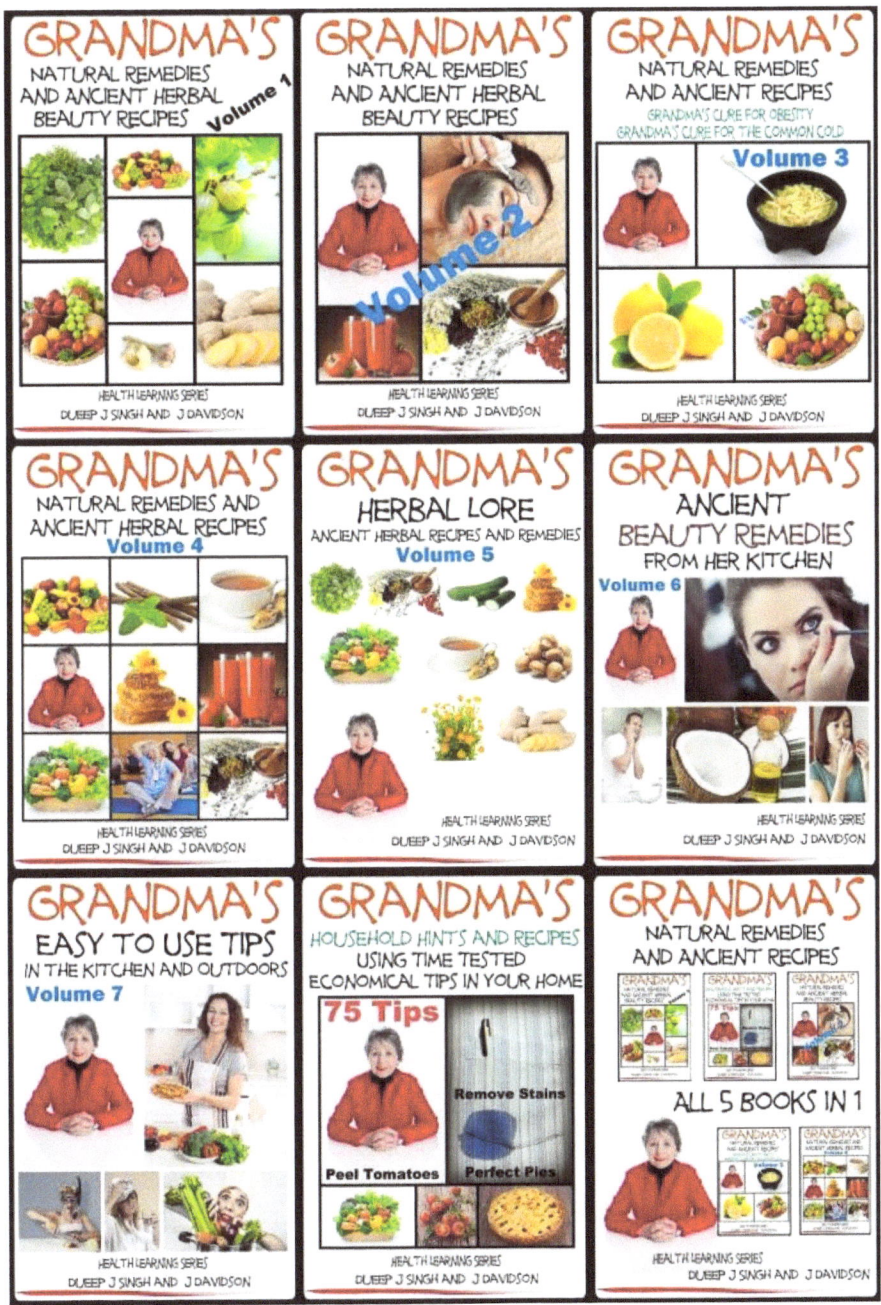

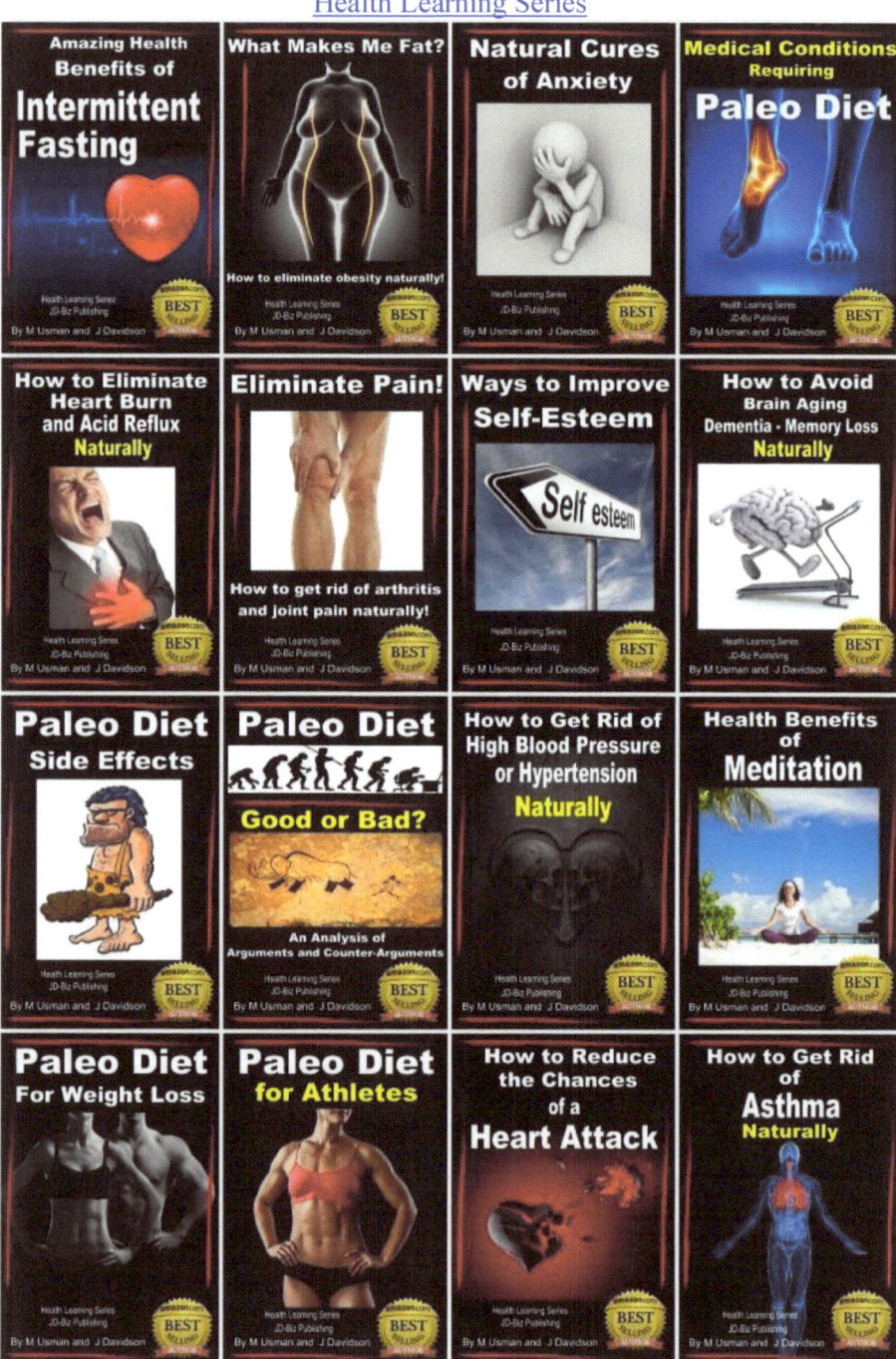

Amazing Animal Book Series

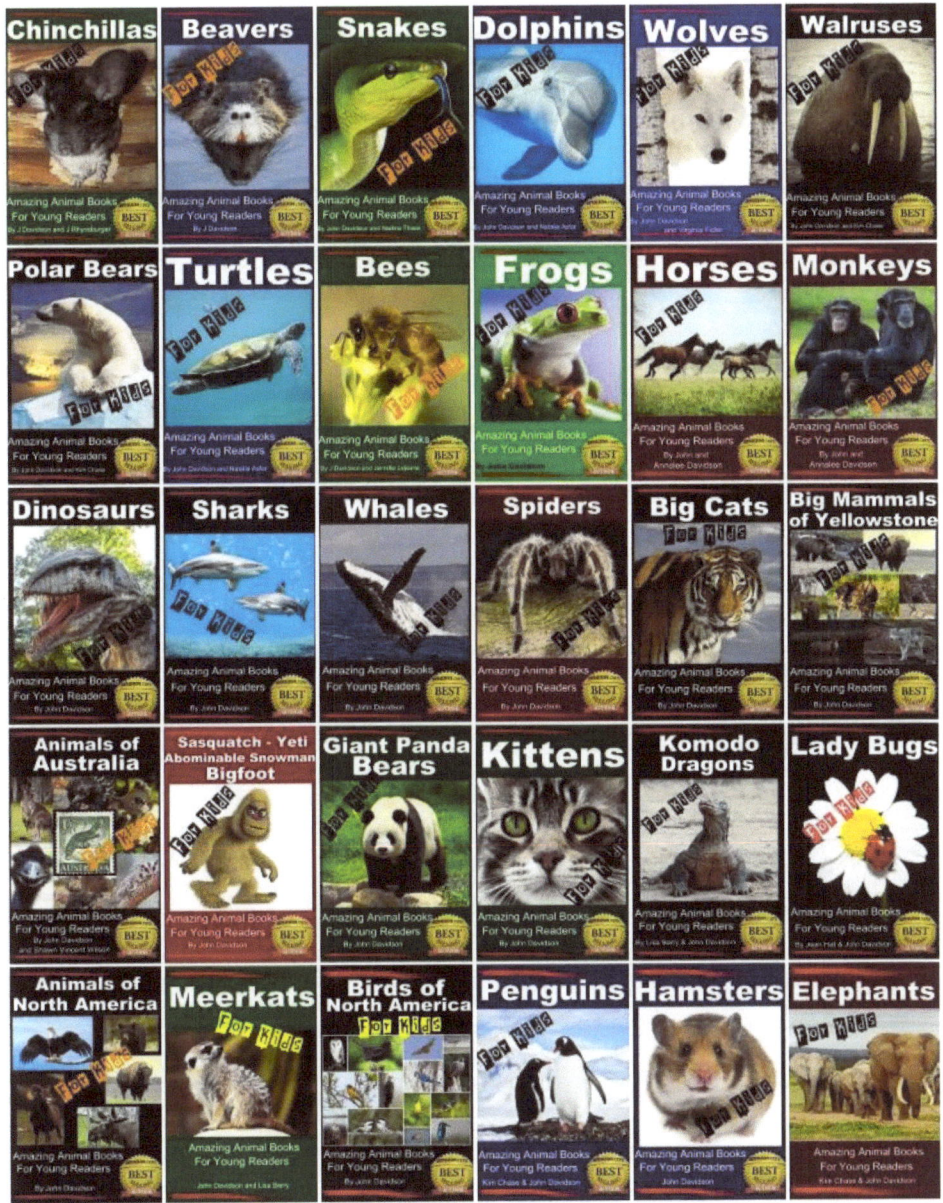

Learn To Draw Series

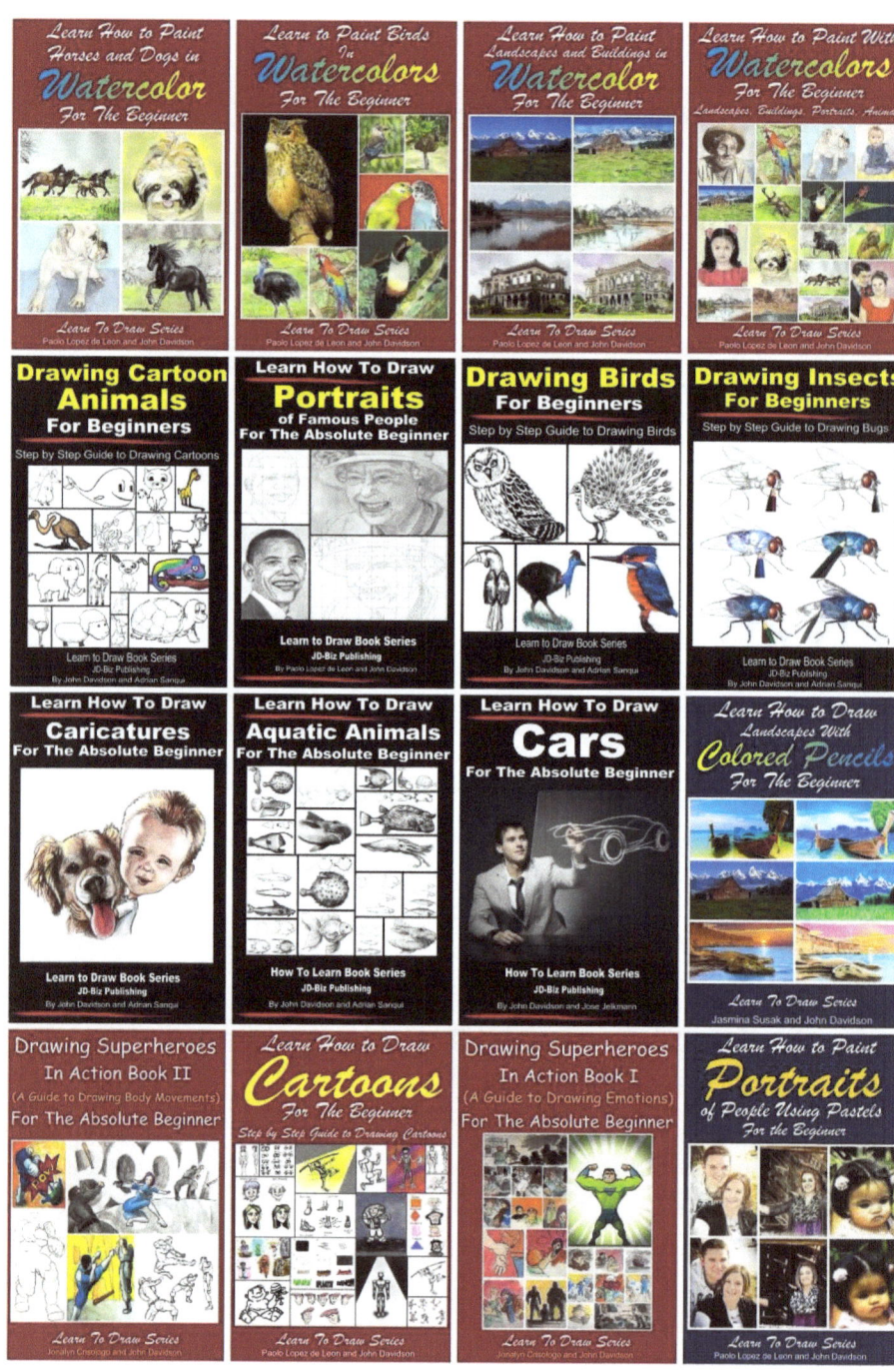

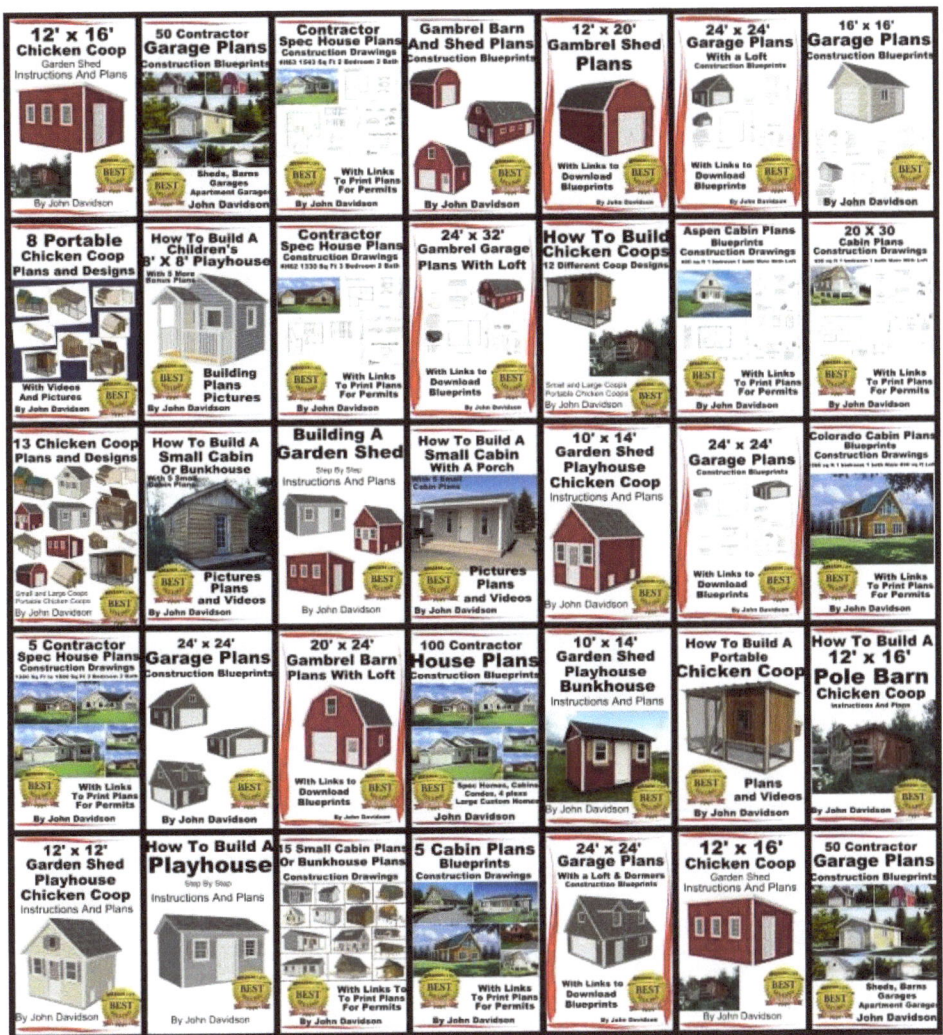

Entreprenleur Book Series

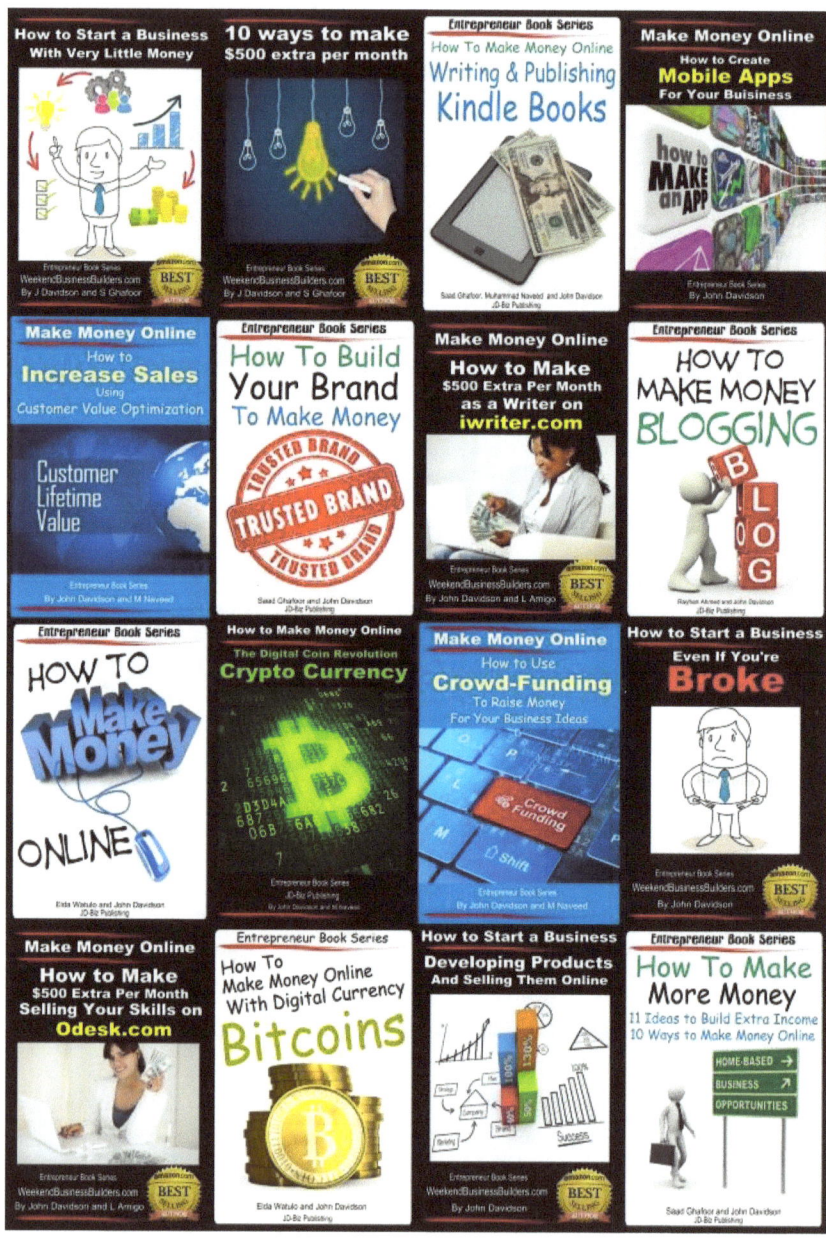

Our books are available at

1. Amazon.com

2. Barnes and Noble

3. Itunes

4. Kobo

5. Smashwords

6. Google Play Books

Download Free Books!

http://MendonCottageBooks.com

Publisher

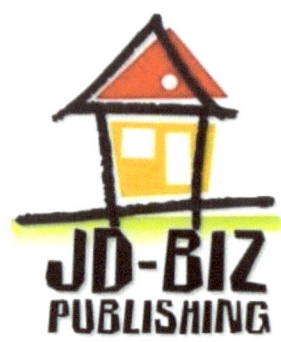

JD-Biz Corp

P O Box 374

Mendon, Utah 84325

http://www.jd-biz.com/

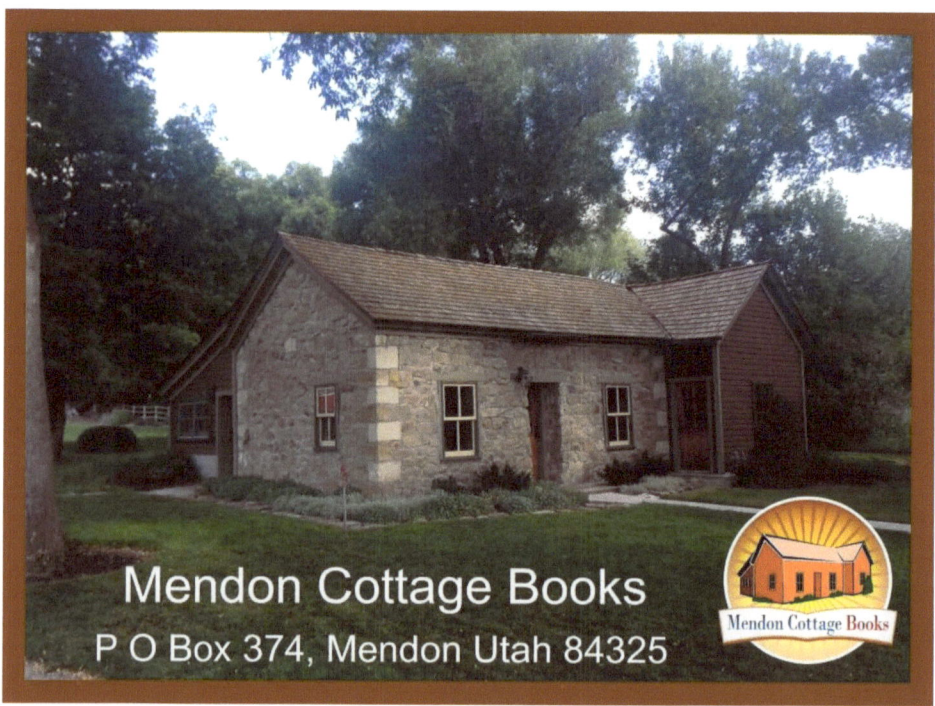